# Differential Diagnosis in Small Animal Cytology

## The Skin and Subcutis

# Differential Diagnosis in Small Animal Cytology

## The Skin and Subcutis

Francesco Cian

and

Paola Monti

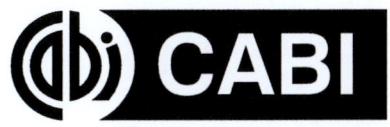

CABI is a trading name of CAB International

| | |
|---|---|
| CABI | CABI |
| Nosworthy Way | 745 Atlantic Avenue |
| Wallingford | 8th Floor |
| Oxfordshire OX10 8DE | Boston, MA 02111 |
| UK | USA |

Tel: +44 (0)1491 832111
Fax: +44 (0)1491 833508
E-mail: info@cabi.org
Website: www.cabi.org

Tel: +1 (617)682-9015
E-mail: cabi-nao@cabi.org

A catalogue record for this book is available from the British Library, London, UK.

Library of Congress Cataloging-in-Publication Data

Names: Cian, Francesco, author. | Monti, Paola (Consultant veterinary clinical pathologist), author. | C.A.B. International, issuing body.
Title: Differential diagnosis in small animal cytology : the skin and subcutis / Francesco Cian and Paola Monti.
Description: Oxfordshire, UK ; Boston, MA : CABI, [2019] | Includes bibliographical references and index.
Identifiers: LCCN 2019013159 (print) | LCCN 2019014194 (ebook) | ISBN 9781786392268 (ePDF) | ISBN 9781786392275 (ePub) | ISBN 9781786392251 (pbk : alk. paper)
Subjects: | MESH: Dog Diseases--diagnosis | Skin Diseases--veterinary | Cat Diseases--diagnosis | Cytodiagnosis--veterinary | Diagnosis, Differential | Pets
Classification: LCC SF992.S55 (ebook) | LCC SF992.S55 C53 2019 (print) | NLM SF 992.S55 | DDC 636.089/075--dc23
LC record available at https://lccn.loc.gov/2019013159

ISBN-13: 978 1 78639 225 1 (paperback)
      978 1 78639 226 8 (ePDF)
      978 1 78639 227 5 (ePub)

Commissioning Editor: Alex Lainsbury
Editorial Assistant: Emma McCann
Production Editor: Kate Hill

Typeset by SPi, Pondicherry, India
Printed and bound by CPI Group (UK) Ltd, Croydon, CR0 4YY

'When we read, we are not looking for new ideas, but to see our own thoughts given the seal of confirmation on the printed page. The words that strike us are those that awake an echo in a zone we have already made our own – the place where we live – and the vibration enables us to find fresh starting points within ourselves.'

*'Leggendo non cerchiamo idee nuove, ma pensieri già da noi pensati, che acquistano sulla pagina un suggello di conferma. Ci colpiscono degli altri le parole che risuonano in una zona già nostra – che già viviamo – e facendola vibrare ci permettono di cogliere nuovi spunti dentro di noi.'*

Cesare Pavese,
***Il mestiere di vivere: Diario 1935–1950***

# Contents

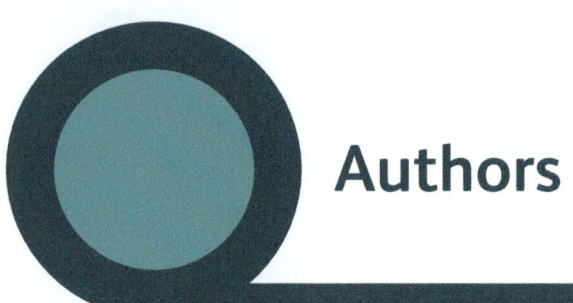

# Authors

**Francesco Cian** DVM, DipECVCP, FRCPath, MRCVS
Email: francesco.cian@hotmail.it

Francesco qualified from University of Padua (Italy) with a DVM in 2006 and spent the next 4 years in small animal practice. In 2010, he started a residency programme in Clinical Pathology at the University of Cambridge, which he finished in 2013, attaining both an ECVCP and FRCPath diploma. Francesco joined the Animal Health Trust (AHT) in 2013 as Head of Clinical Pathology, and since September 2015 he has been working for Battlab (LABOKLIN). Francesco has a special interest in lymphoproliferative disorders of dogs and cats and flow cytometry.

He is member of the cytology examination committee of the European College of Veterinary Clinical Pathology (ECVCP) and is author of several publications in peer-reviewed journals. He co-authored with Paola Monti the cytology chapter of the third edition of the *BSAVA Manual of Veterinary Clinical Pathology* and is editor of the second edition of *Veterinary Cytology: Dog, Cat, Horse and Cow: Self-Assessment Color Review* (CRC Press).

**Paola Monti** DVM, MSc, FRCPath, DipACVP (Clinical Pathology), MRCVS
Email: paolamonti@hotmail.com

Paola qualified from University of Bologna (Italy) with a DVM in 2002. In 2005 she moved to the UK where she spent the first years in small animal practice. In 2008, she started a Royal College of Veterinary Surgeons (RCVS) Trust funded residency programme in clinical pathology at the University of Cambridge. After her training, she obtained both the ACVP and FRCPath diplomas in clinical pathology and in 2015 she received the RCVS Specialist Status in clinical pathology.

Since 2012, Paola has been working at DWR Diagnostic as a clinical pathologist consultant. She has a special interest in cytology and laboratory quality management. She is an examiner of the Royal College of Pathologists (RCPath), author of several publications in peer-reviewed journals and co-author of the cytology and quality assurance chapters of the third edition of the *BSAVA Manual of Veterinary Clinical Pathology.*

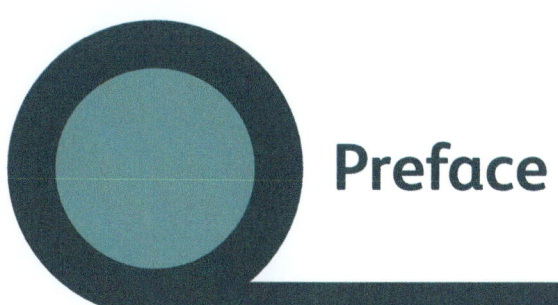

# Preface

Having worked with both the authors, who are internationally renowned veterinary clinical pathologists, I can attest to their incredible passion for cytology, constant thirst for new knowledge and strong attention to detail. Thanks to all these qualities and the authors' extensive diagnostic experience, the readers can benefit from a book designed as both written text and an atlas to provide an up-to-date guide to the cytological diagnosis of cutaneous and subcutaneous diseases of small animals. The authors did an extraordinary job in integrating their wealth of knowledge on the topics with practical competency, reviewing their work and summarizing the information in a reader-friendly and schematic format.

The book is divided into two parts. The first part provides general information on how to prepare and read a cytological specimen and this information is vital for students, veterinary practitioners and residents who approach for the first time the cytology of the skin and subcutis. The first part of the book also includes a chapter dedicated to the choice and use of the microscope, written in collaboration with Ian Baldwin, sales director of a microscope company and expert in the field.

The second part of the book describes the most cytologically relevant canine and feline diseases of the skin and subcutis. I am sure this will represent an extremely valuable resource for clinical pathologists, including experienced diagnosticians. The conditions are covered in a comprehensive and detailed manner, taking into account the improved understanding on pathogenesis and anatomical structure of origin of the lesions and using the most up-to-date terminology and classification schemes. In this second part of the book a great emphasis is placed on the description of the cellular morphology, supported by over 100 original images, and distinguishing features of the various conditions as the basis of an accurate cytological interpretation and formulation of a differential diagnosis. Details of disease incidence, clinical presentation and biological behaviour are also given in the text and the information becomes an amazing tool available for diagnosticians to produce report comments.

In conclusion, this book is an excellent benchside reference for those interested in understanding, interpreting and reporting canine and feline cytology of the skin and subcutis.

**Roberta Rasotto**
DVM, PhD, Dipl.ECVP, MRCVS
EBVS® and RCVS Specialist in Veterinary Pathology

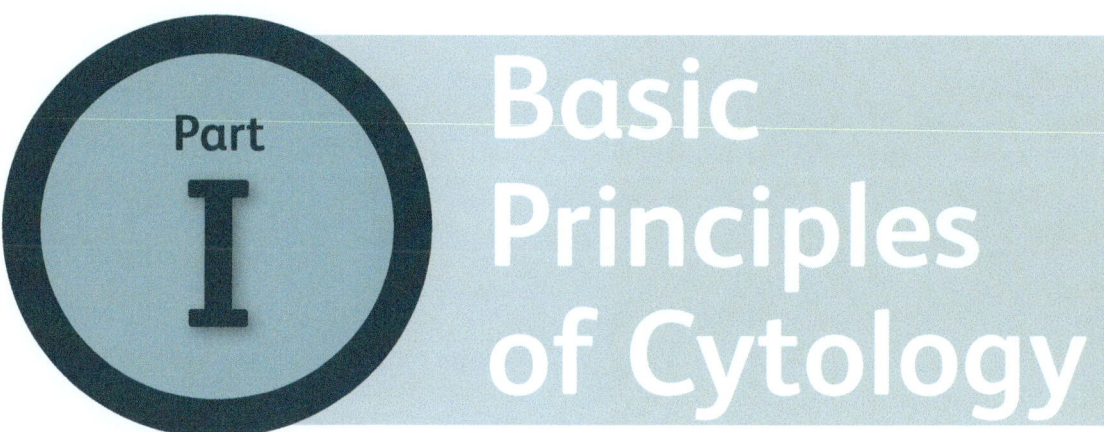

# Part I

# Basic Principles of Cytology

# 1 Guide to the Choice and Correct Use of the Microscope

## (Ian Baldwin)

The optical microscope is as important to the pathologist now as it was 100 years ago (and surprisingly still similar in function and use). Choosing an instrument of the correct quality, specification, construction and support is vital for obtaining good quality images, ensuring ease and comfort of use and maintaining the microscope over the career-life of the pathologist. The pathologist should have a fundamental knowledge of:

- How to set up a microscope to obtain the best images.
- How to keep the instrument in good condition.

The aim of this chapter is to give a practical pointer as to the type of microscope to purchase, what to look for, the questions to ask the supplier, and some tips on everyday use and care.

Everything in this guide refers to the upright or compound microscope. There are other types of microscopes, such as dissecting or operating microscopes, and most of the information discussed here is applicable to these as well. However, there are specific technical differences that will not be covered. This chapter will be focused on the basic brightfield technique used for examining stained specimens on glass slides.

## 1.1 Choosing a Supplier

Purchasing a microscope is much like any other large capital purchase, be it a television or a car. Although different models are available, it is better to purchase from the supplier that provides the best information, seems the most knowledgeable on the product and offers the most comprehensive after-sales support. Aspects to look for when purchasing a microscope should include the following:

- Installation and training: is this provided by the supplier?
- Length and level of cover of the warranty.
- Telephone/email support: is there a specialist at the supplier's office who can be contacted for help or an area representative who can call or visit to assist?

## 1.2 Parts of a Microscope

### Microscope head
There are four types of microscope heads:

- Monocular.
- Binocular.
- Trinocular.
- Ergonomic.

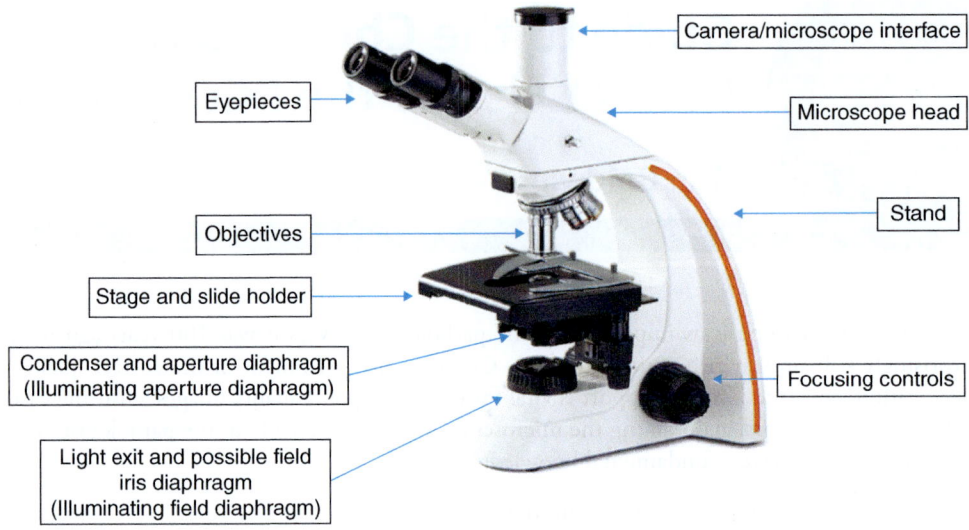

**Fig. 1.1.** Structure of a light microscope.

Monocular head microscopes are very low-cost instruments and are not comfortable for long-term use. Therefore, a binocular head is considered a minimum requirement. A trinocular tube is required if there is the need to add a camera to the microscope.

The ergonomic head allows users of different height to adjust the head angle in order to achieve the most comfortable and safe viewing angle for prolonged microscope use.

## Microscope stand

The microscope stand nearly always has a coaxial coarse and fine focusing mechanism. The illumination system can be integrated within the stand or located in a lamp-house at the back of the microscope. More sophisticated stands, usually designed for clinical use, have a low-position stage and focusing controls, in order to guarantee reduced hand and wrist fatigue. Some stands are also equipped with an adjustable focus height safety lock, which can be set to avoid hitting the slide into the objective, thus destroying the specimen and potentially damaging the objective lenses.

There are two mechanically different versions of microscope stands, which require two different means of setting up the components. These are differentiated based on their type of illumination and are as follows:

- **Koehler illumination microscopes**
  These clinical/research-grade microscopes generate an extremely even illumination of the sample, ensuring that an image of the light source (e.g. halogen lamp filament or LED light) is not visible in the resulting image.

- **Critical illumination microscopes**
  These lower-cost systems rely on frosted glass diffusers. The major problem associated with this type of microscope is the evenness of illumination, as an image of the illumination source is visible in the resulting image.

## Eyepieces

The microscope is invariably supplied with a pair of 10× eyepieces (other magnifications such as 15× are rarely offered as an option). The magnification power is recorded on every eyepiece, followed by another number. The designations might look like the following:

- 10×/20
- WF (widefield) 10/22
- WF 10×/22

The number (e.g. /20) following the power of magnification of the eyepiece (e.g. 10×) represents the field-of-view number, or field number, and it designates the size of the visual field (measured in millimetres) provided by any given objective. The larger the number, the larger is the field of view of the specimen. It is not recommended to purchase a microscope with a field of view less than 20 mm; ideally, a field of view of 22 mm guarantees a comfortable image with sufficient coverage of the specimen. Some of the eyepieces may also display an image of a pair of glasses. This indicates that they are *high-eyepoint*, designed to be comfortable when used wearing spectacles. Some of the eyepieces allow the insertion of a measurement scale (eyepiece scale, reticule or graticule).

## Objectives

There are several different types and special variants of objectives. These can be broadly classified based on their qualities as:

- Achromatic: routine quality.
- Fluorite: research/clinical grade.
- Apochromatic: highest possible quality and resolution.

The quality of an objective depends on the degree of chromatic aberration correction, difference in spherical aberration and numerical aperture.

Understanding the specifications displayed on the objective is very important to ensure the correct use of the lens. The key elements of an objective and the identification of the technical points specified on the barrel are discussed below.

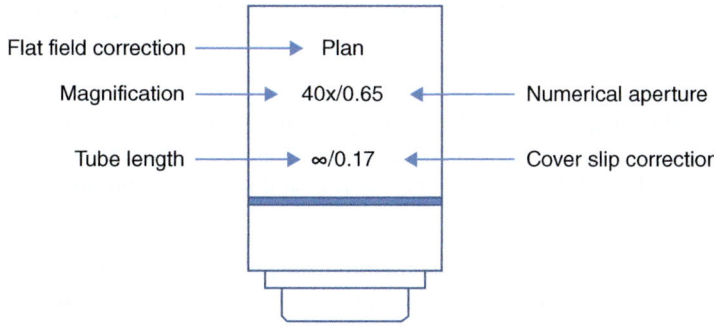

**Fig. 1.2.** Microscope objective.

- **Plan**
  Very low-cost microscopes or teaching microscopes have objectives that are not guaranteed to give a flat field. In these cases, the borders of the field might look slightly blurry. An objective guaranteed to be flat-field is defined as *plan, plano* or just *PL*.

- **Magnification**
  This represents the magnification of the objective and, multiplied by the eyepiece magnification (most likely 10×), gives the magnification to the eyes. Therefore, a 40× objective with 10× eyepieces gives a total magnification of 400× to the eyes. The most common objectives used in biological microscopes are 4×, 10×, 20×, 40×/50× and 100×.

- **Numerical aperture**
  This is a technical term and allows the calculation of the resolution of the objective. It represents the ability to gather light and resolve fine specimen details at a fixed object distance. High-quality objectives (in order: achromatic–fluorite–apochromatic) have a larger numerical aperture guaranteeing a better resolution of the image. To reach a numerical aperture of 1 or above, the objective must be an immersion objective.

- **Tube length**
  This is a technical aspect of the optical design. Lower-quality and older models have a fixed tube length, usually 160 mm. Modern microscopes have an infinity-corrected tube length. This is not related with quality but allows insertion of accessories between the body and the head (e.g. dual viewing tube), without changing the magnification of the image to the eyes. Using both fixed tube-length and infinity objectives on the same microscope will cause very poor images and risks damaging the objectives.

- **Cover slip correction**
  The vast majority of dry objectives of 20× magnification and above are designed to be used with a standard cover slip over the specimen and the cover slip acts as a lens. If the cover slip is not in place, the image will not be as good. The thickness of a standard cover slip is 0.17 mm.

As discussed above, in order to get the highest numerical aperture and resolution, immersion oil is used between the objective and the specimen. If an objective is designed for oil immersion use, the word *Oil* will be written on the barrel of the objective, after the magnification/numerical aperture (e.g. Plan 100×/1.25 Oil). The choice of good-quality oil is essential, as it determines the quality of the image. Different oils should never be mixed, as they may react and increase the turbidity of the oil. The use of old, low-cost or especially viscous yellow oil should also be avoided.

If a dry objective (e.g. 40×) is contaminated with immersion oil, this can be cleaned off by using a mild solvent (e.g. 30% ethanol) or with a commercially available cleaning solution for camera lenses.

## Condensers

The condenser and its diaphragm (or illuminating aperture) provide a cone of light at the right intensity and angle to ensure the best possible level of resolution of the objective. Depending on the type, condensers have different levels of correction and numerical apertures (NA). The most common condensers are:

- Abbe condenser: this concentrates and controls the light that passes through the specimen prior to entering the objective and has no optical corrections. It has two controls, one which moves the Abbe condenser closer to or further from the stage, and another, the iris diaphragm, which controls the diameter of the beam of light. The controls can be used to optimize brightness, evenness of illumination, and contrast. The Abbe condenser is adequate for most brightfield applications, however, its limitation comes when using high magnification objectives.

- Achromatic and aplanatic condensers: an aplanatic condenser corrects for spherical aberration in the concentrated light path, while an achromatic compound condenser corrects for both spherical and chromatic aberrations. This helps to achieve an optimum resolution and highest potential numerical NA from a microscope.

For the routine clinical microscope, an Abbe 0.9 is considered adequate and is normally present on most standard microscopes. More advanced microscopes with fluorite objectives usually carry a higher-corrected condenser.

## Microscope illumination

For a very long time, microscopes were equipped with tungsten–halogen filament lamps. The only disadvantage of these lamps was the short lifespan caused by the high temperatures reached when in use. Over the past few years, microscopes have moved to LED illumination, giving a bright white light without heat dissipation. However, the colour characteristics of LED lights are not directly comparable to halogen lights, especially with earlier LED illumination. For this reason, an adaptation time is recommended when changing from halogen to LED lighting, as the appearance of some stains may look different depending on the light source.

# 1.3 Setting up a Microscope

There is only one way a microscope should be set up for any given objective. Deviating from this will only reduced the quality of the image. When setting up a microscope it is important to carry out the following:

- Position the condenser to the correct height and centration in relation to the objective.
- Ensure that the diaphragm (or diaphragms) on the microscope is correctly set (see later).

## Eyepieces

Often overlooked, the eyepieces need to be correctly set or eyestrain will occur. Most microscopes have one eyepiece with a focusing capability and markings showing + and − dioptre settings.

**Procedure**
- Focus on a specimen looking through the fixed, non-adjustable eyepiece.
- Looking through the adjustable eyepiece, rotate this until the focus is reached (sharp image).

## Illumination
- **Koehler illumination**

**Procedure**
- Place a slide with a good contrast specimen on the stage and use the 10× objective. Focus on the specimen with the focus controls.
- Move the condenser using the condenser rack and pinion controls under the stage until it is about 0.5 cm from the top.
- Close the field diaphragm. At this point the leaves of the diaphragm (which may not be in the centre of the field) will become visible.
- Move the condenser up and down until the leaves are in focus.
- Use a knurled screw or Allen key (usually in the front of the condenser mount, at the left or right) to centre the image of the diaphragm.
- Open the field diaphragm until it is just out of the field of view.

In this way the condenser will be at the correct height and centred in the optical pathway, allowing the best illumination of the specimen to achieve the best possible image quality.

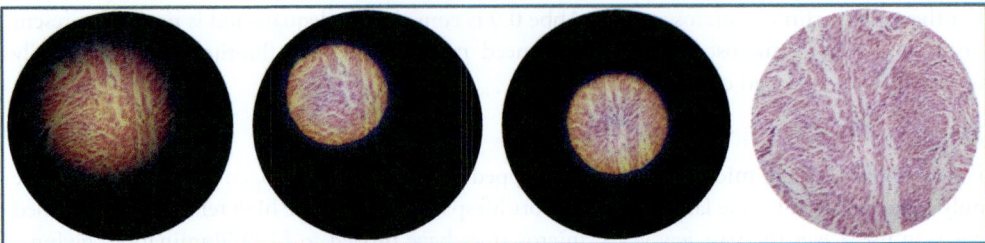

**Fig. 1.3.** Adjustment of Koehler illumination system.

- **Critical illumination**

  This procedure is more difficult because there is no field diaphragm in the focused image. The illuminating aperture diaphragm (condenser diaphragm for ease of terminology) should be used instead. This is not usually visible. It becomes visible by removing an eyepiece and looking into the tube (keeping a distance of 10–15 cm from the tube).

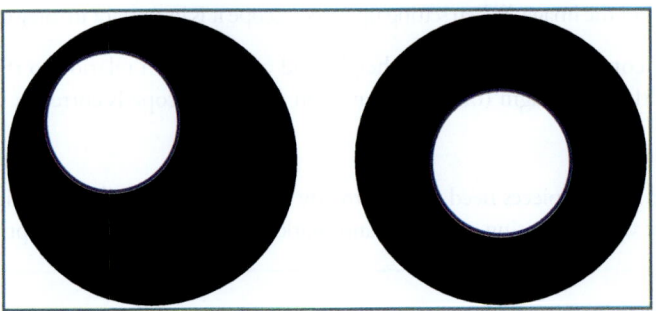

**Fig. 1.4.** Adjustment of critical illumination system.

**Procedure**
- Focus on a specimen on the stage and raise the condenser to the top, or very near the top of travel.
- Remove one eyepiece and look into the tube until only the edges of the condenser diaphragm become visible but not the image of the specimen.
- Centre the condenser using the front-facing centration screws on the condenser.

## Condenser diaphragm

This is considered one of the most important parts of the setting up of a microscope. If the condenser diaphragm is too closed, the resolution of the image decreases significantly. The practical problem with this type of diaphragm is that the correct set for a lower magnification (e.g. 10× objective) is too closed for a higher magnification. This means that the condenser diaphragm should be opened when going up with the objectives.

The condenser adjusts the cone of light entering the objective. It also ensures that not too much light is focused on the specimen by lowering the contrast through glare. If it is too closed, the resolution of the image will be limited.

> **Procedure**
> • Look at a specimen in focus and open the condenser diaphragm fully.
> • Gently close the condenser until the light just starts to decrease.

A good microscope will have the correct condenser position marked on it, so it is possible to know exactly where to set the lever.

## 1.4  Care of the Microscope

In general, modern microscopes require very little maintenance. The key care point for a microscope is to keep it covered when not in use, as dust is the great enemy of optical microscopes.

The other major problem is the contamination of dry objectives with immersion oil object-ives. The more modern and sophisticated objectives have a flat front end, which is easy to clean. Older objectives are concave, making cleaning much more difficult. It is important to follow the microscope manufacturer's advice on what cleaning agent to use. If unknown, a dilute ethanol solution or proprietary camera lens solution can be used.

## 1.5  Taking Pictures of Microscope Images

There are two main types of camera systems than can be used: dedicated, and commercial digital single-lens reflex (DSLR).

### Dedicated microscope camera

The advantage of using this type of camera is that it provides a full-screen live image at full (or selectable) resolution with many controls for setting the parameters, such as white balance and correct exposure. This allows the user to see exactly what is being captured by the camera. Moreover, nearly all microscope cameras are equipped with comprehensive software, including advanced processing capabilities, calibrated manual measurements and scale bars. The only downside is that most microscope cameras need a computer to run. However, the market also offers high definition multi-media interface (HDMI)-enabled cameras, which run straight out to a monitor, have integral set-up and control software and capture the image to an integral standard SD card. These cameras also have very fast frame rates and are particularly good for teaching/discussion applications with a seamless live image.

### Commercial DSLR camera

Most modern DSLR cameras do have some form of output to a television screen or live to a personal computer. The images obtained can be very good but these cameras require much more user input to get correct and reproducible results. A major point about using a DSLR is that a good-quality interface to the microscope is required and incurs an add-itional cost.

## The camera/microscope interface

To get good results is important to use the correct interface between the microscope and the camera. The majority of dedicated microscope cameras use a so-called *C mount* interface. C mounts come with different magnification factors, typically 1×/0.5×/0.4×/0.35×.

Early cameras had very large sensors and a 1× C mount was adequate to guarantee a large visual field. However, camera sensors have become smaller over time, leading to a highly magnified and consequently very small proportion of visual field presented to the camera sensor. For this reason, reduction lenses are required.

# 2 Collection, Preparation and Staining of Cytology Specimens

## 2.1 Materials

- Needles (21–25G) and syringes (2–10 ml) for fine-needle sampling of cutaneous and subcutaneous masses with/without aspiration.
- Cotton swabs, ideally dampened with saline, for swab sampling.
- Glass slides, possibly with frosted end for ease of labelling and identification.
- Plain and EDTA tubes for fluid specimens (e.g. cystic, fluid-filled lesions, abscesses, etc.) for culture and cytology, respectively. The EDTA sample is not suitable for culture, due to its bacteriostatic effect.
- Slide holders to protect smears from breakage when sent to an external laboratory for evaluation.

## 2.2 Sampling Techniques

### Fine-needle sampling with aspiration

- **Advantages**
  Suitable for sampling most skin lesions, especially those with poor tendency to exfoliate (e.g. mesenchymal proliferations).
- **Disadvantages**
  The excessive negative pressure applied during the process may cause cellular damage, especially of more fragile cell types (e.g. lymphoid cells). Excessive haemodilution of the sample may also occur.
- **Technique**
  Connect the needle to the syringe. Insert the needle within the mass. Apply suction and redirect the needle multiple times. Discontinue suction before withdrawal. Detach the syringe and draw in some air. Reattach the syringe to needle and expel the sampled material on to labelled glass slides.

### Fine-needle sampling without aspiration

- **Advantages**
  Suitable for sampling skin lesions with good tendency to exfoliate. This technique better preserves the morphology of fragile cells and minimizes blood contamination.
- **Disadvantages**
  May yield an insufficient cell harvest from poorly exfoliative masses.
- **Technique**
  Insert the needle within the mass and re-direct it multiple times in different areas of the lesion. Withdraw the needle, attach the syringe containing some air and expel the material on to labelled glass slides.

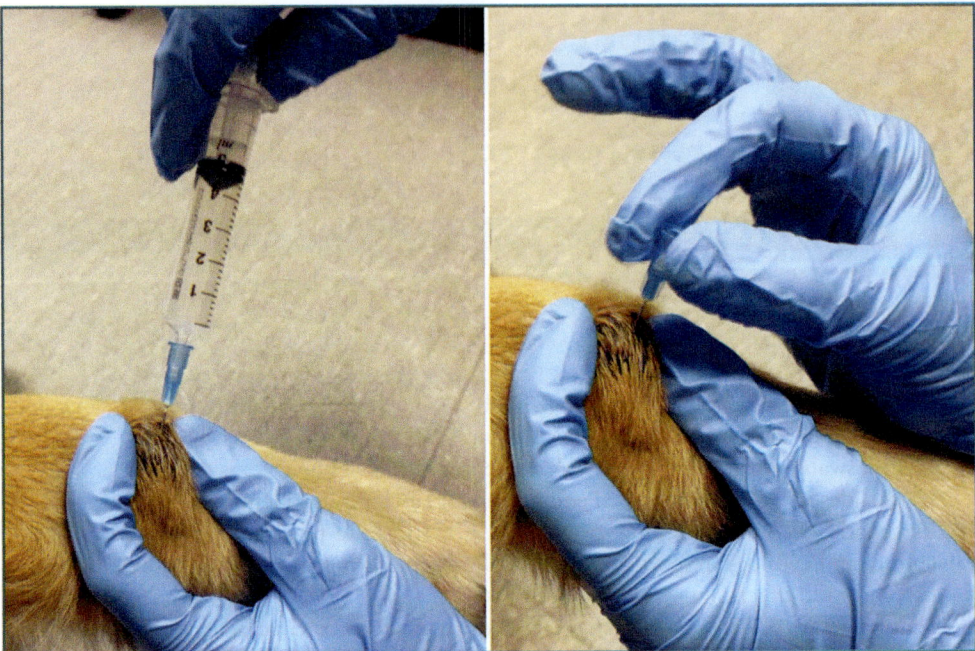

**Fig. 2.1.** Fine-needle sampling technique: with (left) and without (right) aspiration.

## Imprint

- **Advantages**
  Appropriate for ulcerated, wet, thin lesions, which are not suitable for fine needle aspiration.

- **Disadvantages**
  The sample obtained is only representative of the superficial part of the lesion.

- **Technique**
  Gently blot the tissue of interest with a sterile gauze to remove surface blood. Touch the surface of the lesion with the slide.

## Swab

- **Advantages**
  Appropriate for evaluation of cavities, sinus tracts and draining lesions (e.g. ear swabs, vaginal swabs).

- **Technique**
  Insert the swab inside the sinus tract or draining lesion. Extract the swab and roll it along the slide.

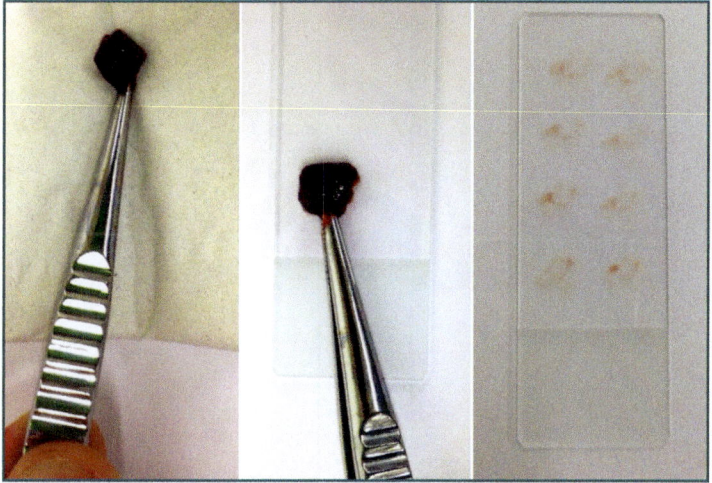

**Fig. 2.2.** Impression smear technique.

## 2.3 Smear Preparation Techniques

### Squash preparation

- **Use**

  Appropriate for most cytology samples.

- **Technique**

  The material obtained by fine-needle sampling (with or without syringe) is expelled on to a slide. A second smear is placed on the top of the first slide in order to allow spreading of the material. The slides are then pulled apart, resulting in cells smearing on both slides. Care should be taken not to apply excessive pressure, which may result in cell damage. The sample material should not travel over the edge of the smear.

### Blood smear technique

- **Use**

  Appropriate for slide preparation of liquid samples.

- **Technique**

  A drop of specimen is placed at the end of a slide. The end of a second slide is placed in front of the drop at approximately an angle of 30–45 degrees and slid backwards until it comes into contact with the sample drop. The sample will spread out along the width of the spreader slide. The spreader slide is advanced forwards, creating a smear with a feathered edge.

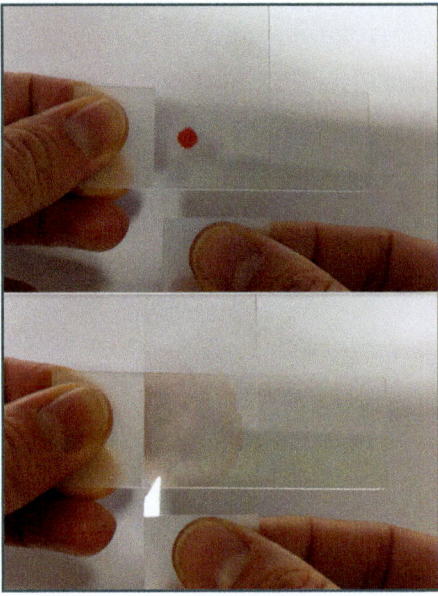

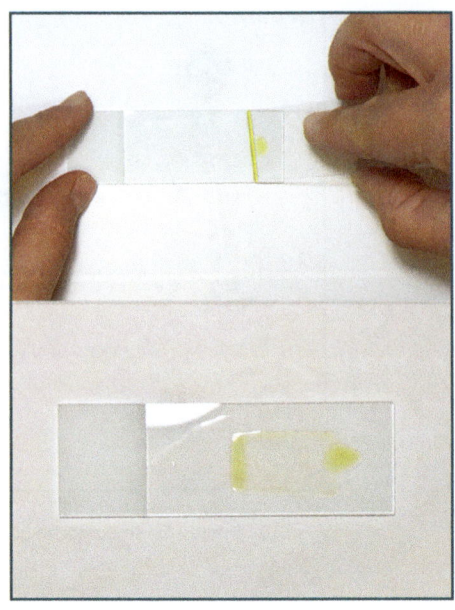

**Fig. 2.3.** Squash smear preparation.

**Fig. 2.4.** Blood smear technique.

## Line smear technique

*   **Use**

    Appropriate for hypocellular fluids.
*   **Technique**

    The procedure is similar to the blood smear technique, but instead of completing the smear, the spreader slide is lifted vertically prior to formation of a feathered edge. This results in concentration of cells along a 'line' where the smear is interrupted.

## Centrifugation

*   **Use**

    Appropriate for cytology preparation of hypocellular fluids.
*   **Technique**

    Concentration may be obtained by cytocentrifugation or traditional low-speed centrifugation. The latter requires a drop of the sediment to be transferred on to a slide and then smeared with either the squash or blood smear technique, depending on its density.

## 2.4 Slide Staining

Stains most commonly used for routine skin cytology are Romanowsky type stains; these include rapid (e.g. Diff-Quik®) and Wright-Giemsa stains. Staining protocols may differ according to the manufacturer. Note: before staining, slides should be rapidly air-dried.

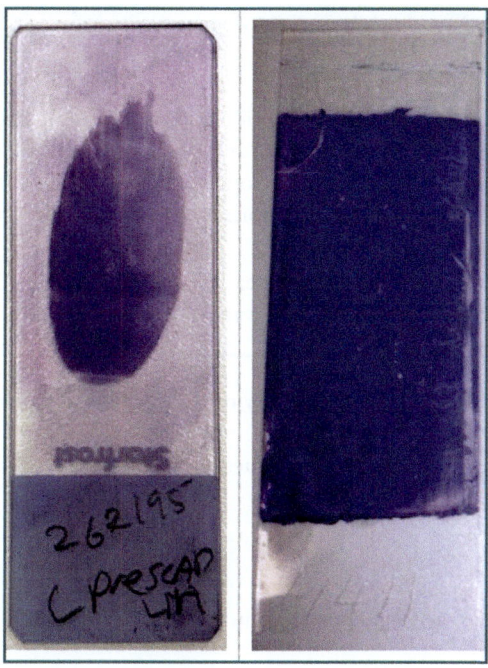

**Fig. 2.5.** Cytology slides. The slide on the left shows an ideal cytological preparation. The material is nicely distributed on the slide, which has the classic ovoid-shaped appearance. The slide on the right is considered suboptimal: it is not properly labelled and it is too thick because of an excessive amount of material present on the slide and insufficient smearing.

# 3  Guidelines to Cytology Smear Examination

A correct approach to slide examination is considered crucial for an appropriate interpretation of cytological samples and to reduce the chances of missing important details. A poor and superficial examination technique may lead to a wrong diagnosis and incorrect clinical decisions. Therefore, cytological evaluation should be performed with a systematic approach, conducted in the same way each time a slide is examined.

The overall accuracy of cytology testing greatly depends on the quality of the specimen, including the cellularity of the sample, the preservation of the cells and the quality of the staining.

> **Factors that can have an impact on the quality of the cytological specimens and may result in a non-diagnostic sample**
> - Inadequate sampling or smearing technique.
> - Excessive suction.
> - Traumatic smearing.
> - Haemorrhagic lesions.
> - Aspiration from a necrotic centre.
> - Poorly exfoliative lesions (e.g. lesions rich in collagen stroma).
> - Staining features.
> - Insufficient staining due to incorrect procedure or old stains.
> - Sample contamination with lubricant or ultrasound gel.
> - Exposure of the unfixed slides to formalin fumes.

When the aspirates are acellular or mostly contain disrupted cells without a clear and distinct cytoplasm (e.g. bare/naked nuclei), a cytological interpretation may not be possible and re-sampling should be recommended. Similarly, if the sample is adequately cellular and the cells are intact but the staining quality is poor, a cytological diagnosis might be precluded.

# 3.1 Step-by-step Approach to the Slide Examination and Description

## Step 1: Low-power magnification (4×, 10×, 20×)

Smears should initially be scanned with low-power objectives to gain an appreciation of the overall cellularity and cell preservation. It is important to examine the entire smear, including the feathered edges.

The following points should be considered when examining a cytology smear at low magnification:

- Is the cellularity adequate for the type of specimen and collection technique? Is it enough to attempt a diagnosis?
- Are the cells adequately stained and well preserved?
- Is there any non-cellular background material that may be of significance, such as matrix, cytoplasmic fragments (lymphoglandular bodies), etc?
- Is there a monomorphic or a mixed population of nucleated cells? Are these homogenously distributed throughout the smear?
- Is there evidence of any typical cell arrangement and/or cytoarchitecture?
- What types of cells are present (e.g. inflammatory cells, tissue cells, or a mixture of the two)?

## Step 2: High-power magnification (40×, 50×, 100×)

High magnification allows for a more detailed evaluation of the cell morphology details.

- **Inflammatory cells**
  The inflammatory process should be classified based on the predominant cell type/types. The morphology of the inflammatory cells should be carefully examined for the presence of significant changes, such as degenerative changes in the neutrophils or phagocytic activity by the macrophages, etc.
- **Infectious agents**
  When appropriate, a thorough examination of the slides for the presence of infectious agents (bacteria, fungi, protozoa, etc.) should be made. Bacteria are usually found in the background of the smears and/or phagocytosed by the neutrophils. Fungi and yeasts are usually found in the background, surrounded by the inflammatory cells, or within macrophages. When a fungal infection is suspected and the aspirates are highly cellular, hyphae are usually hidden amongst the inflammatory cells in the thickest areas of the smear. Protozoa are generally found within macrophages.
- **Tissue cells**
  These can be classified into epithelial, mesenchymal or round cells based on their arrangement and morphology.

  When writing a cytology report, the shape and arrangement of the cells, morphology of the nucleus and cytoplasmic features should be described.
  - Cell type morphology and arrangement:
    - Epithelial cells
    - Shape: cuboidal, polygonal or columnar.
    - Arrangement: cells often exfoliate in cohesive clusters. Their architecture varies depending on the tissue of origin, as illustrated in fig. 3.1.

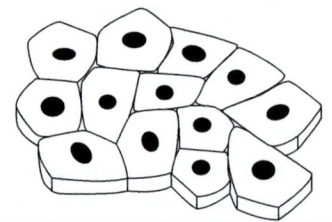 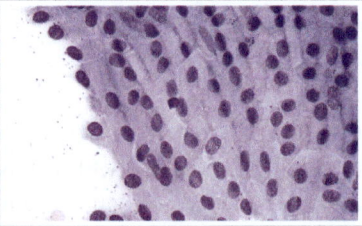

**Pavement**
Cells are flat, polygonal and arranged in thin layers
- Keratinocytes of the superficial layers of the epidermis and superior segment of the hair follicle (infundibulum)
- Squamous cell carcinoma
- Papilloma

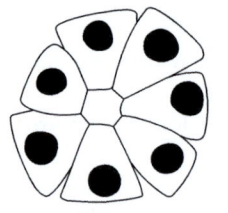 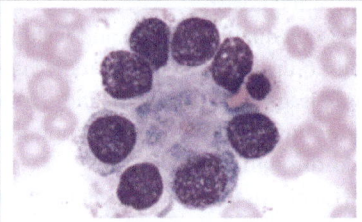

**Acinar**
Cells are cuboidal to columnar and arranged around a central pale area

- Sweat gland tumour
- Anal sac tumour

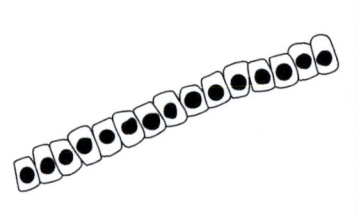 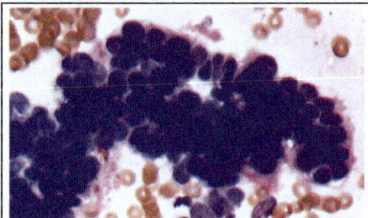

**Palisade**
Cells are cuboidal and arranged in regular rows

- Trichoblastoma
- Basal cell tumour

Ducts may cytologically mimic this type of arrangement (e.g. sweat gland duct adenoma)

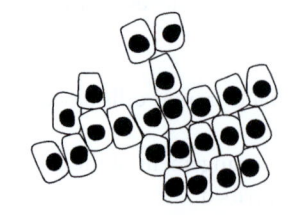 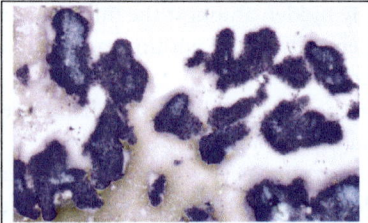

**Trabecular**
Cells are arranged in branching cohesive clusters

- Perianal gland tumour

**Fig. 3.1.** Most common cytoarchitectures that can be found on cytology of cutaneous and subcutaneous lesions. (1) Pavement. (2) Acinar. (3) Palisade. (4) Trabecular. (5) Perivascular. (6) Whorling. (7) Storiform. (*Drawings courtesy of Nic Ilchyshyn, DWR Diagnostic UK.*)

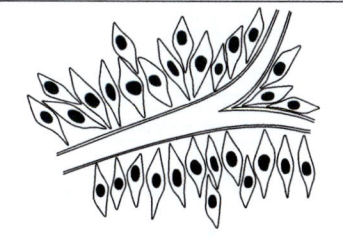 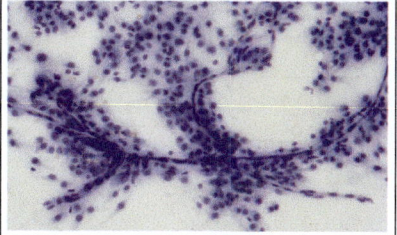

**Perivascular**

Cells are arranged around one or multiple capillaries

- Perivascular wall tumour

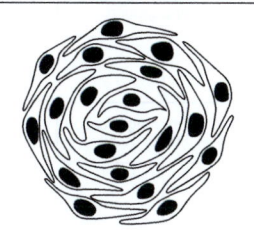 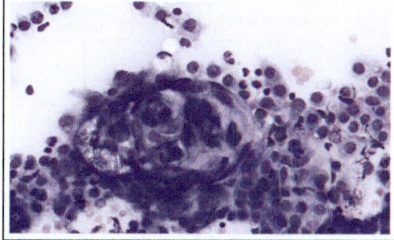

**Whorling**

Cells are whorling around a central small vessel (the vessel is often not seen in this formation)

- Perivascular wall tumour

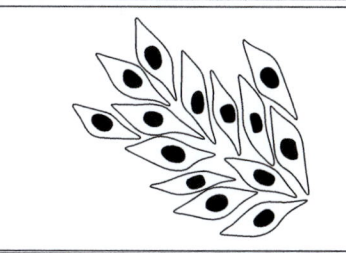 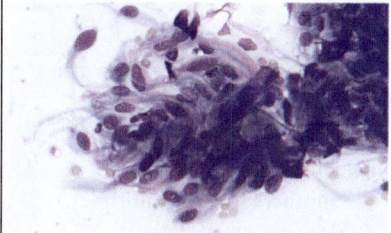

**Storiform**

Cells are spindle shaped and arranged in bundles

- Sarcoma

**Fig. 3.1.** Continued

- Mesenchymal cells:
  - Shape: spindle, fusiform, veiled, stellate, plump-oval.
  - Arrangement: either individual or arranged in non-cohesive aggregates.
- Round cells:
  - Shape: round to oval with well defined margins.
  - Arrangement: cells exfoliate individually.
- Description of the cellular details
  - Nucleus:
    - Shape (e.g. round, oval, irregular).
    - Size (small, medium, large).
    - Location (central, paracentral, eccentric, basal).
    - Chromatin appearance (e.g. finely stippled, granular, coarse, clumped).

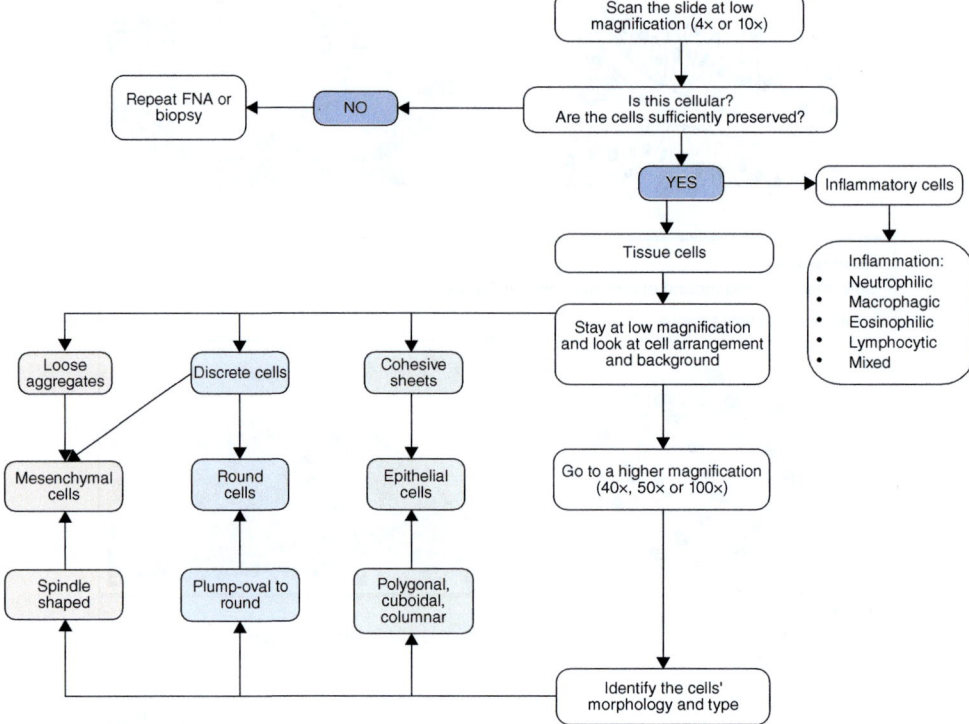

**Fig. 3.2.** Systematic approach to slide examination.

- Nucleolus:
  - Numbers (one or multiple).
  - Size (e.g. small, large).
  - Shape and borders (e.g. round, angular, irregular).
  - Appearance (e.g. inconspicuous, prominent).
- Cytoplasm:
  - Amount (scant, moderate, abundant).
  - Colour (basophilic, eosinophilic, amphophilic, etc.).
  - Texture (smooth, granular, dense, etc.).
  - Content (vacuoles, granules, infectious agents).
  - Borders (distinct, ill-defined).

The slide examination usually continues with the evaluation of criteria of atypia/malignancy (see appropriate section). Malignant tumours usually exfoliate cells that display multiple features of atypia. However, some of these changes may also occur with stimulation of cells associated with hyperplasia, dysplasia or inflammation.

In selected neoplasms (e.g. canine thyroid carcinoma, canine anal sac adenocarcinoma and neuroendocrine tumours), cells can lack significant cytological features of atypia, despite their aggressive behaviour. Other neoplasms, such as cutaneous plasma cell tumour, can display prominent pleomorphism, even if clinically benign. The cytologist should be aware of these exceptions in order to interpret correctly the cytological findings.

## 3.2   Interpretation of the Cytological Findings

Once all slides have been examined and all cell types identified, examined and described and infectious agents identified or ruled out (when possible), all the gathered information should be used to provide a cytological interpretation, preferably contextualized with the clinical presentation and history. For this purpose, the following questions need to be answered:

- What type of process/processes does it likely represent (inflammatory, hyperplastic, dysplastic, neoplastic)?
- If inflammatory, which type of inflammation is present? Can the underlying cause be identified (e.g. infectious agent, foreign material)?
- If neoplastic, can the cell lineage be identified more specifically? Do the cells display or lack features of malignancy?
- What is the degree of confidence of your cytological interpretation? If not definitive, modifiers can be used (e.g. suggestive or supportive of, probable, possible, suspicion for).

### Comment

In a cytology report, the interpretation is followed by a comment, which includes any further information the pathologist feels the need to communicate. This may include an explanation of the interpretation provided, any further test that may be needed to refine the diagnosis, and information about the biological behaviour and prognosis of the disease diagnosed. The following points should be considered during the elaboration of the comment:

- What is the degree of confidence of the interpretation provided?
- Are there additional tests that may be of benefit for confirmation, prognosis, staging or evaluation of the extent of the disease?
- What is the expected biological behaviour based on these findings?

# 4 Cytological Criteria of Malignancy

In tumour cytology, cells are evaluated for the presence of morphological alterations compared with the normal cells from which they originate. When present, these changes are referred to as criteria of malignancy.

In malignant tumours, with the exception of well-differentiated forms and some specific neoplasms, most neoplastic cells show multiple morphological features of atypia. However, some of these changes can also be induced by severe inflammation. For this reason, caution should be exercised in diagnosing neoplasia in the presence of numerous inflammatory cells. In all those cases where a definitive diagnosis is not possible, histopathological examination should be recommended.

The main cytological criteria used to identify malignancy are described in the following sections. Nuclear criteria are considered more significant because they are less likely to be induced by non-neoplastic processes such as inflammation.

## 4.1 General Criteria of Malignancy

- **Arrangement**
  Arrangement is mostly evaluated in epithelial tumours. In non-neoplastic epithelial lesions and in benign epithelial tumours, cells are generally uniformly arranged and mirror the architecture of the normal tissue from which they arise. In malignant tumours, cells undergo an uncontrolled and haphazard growth that can lead to disorganized architectures. Cytologically, this can be observed as *nuclear moulding* (nucleus of one cell to deform around the nucleus of another cell) and *cell crowding* (overlapping of nuclei).
- **Anisocytosis and macrocytosis**
  Anisocytosis (cell size variation) and macrocytosis (presence of exceptionally large cells) should be interpreted in the context of the tissue examined. A mild degree of size variation is considered normal. Moderate to marked anisocytosis is usually considered significant, although this should be interpreted in the context of the characteristics of the tissue of origin.
- **Pleomorphism**
  Pleomorphism is variability in shapes within the same cell type.
- **Loss of cohesion**
  Loss of cohesion is the result of down-regulation of the adhesion cellular molecules. This phenomenon is typically observed in epithelial tumours and is usually associated with increased exfoliation upon aspiration.

## 4.2 Nuclear Criteria

- **Anisokaryosis and macrokaryosis/karyomegaly**
  Anisokaryosis (nuclear size variation) and macrokaryosis/karyomegaly (presence of exceptionally large nuclei) are considered significant when moderate to marked, although this should be interpreted in the context of the characteristics of the tissue of origin.

- **Asynchronous nucleus to cytoplasm maturation**
  A marked variation of this ratio from the normal cell counterpart is considered an abnormal finding.

- **Multinucleation**
  Multinucleation is particularly significant when nuclei within the same cell are variably sized and in the presence of odd numbers of nuclei per cell. Certain non-neoplastic cell types are typically multinucleated (e.g. megakaryocytes, osteoclasts, multinucleated giant inflammatory cells).

- **Nucleoli**
  Nucleoli are nuclear substructures assigned to produce ribosomes and are considered a hallmark of malignancy when they become prominent, multiple, irregularly shaped (e.g. angular, elongated, etc.) and variably sized (anisonucleosis). Some non-neoplastic cells normally contain visible nucleoli (e.g. hepatocytes). Nucleoli may also be spuriously prominent in cells that are either ruptured or under-stained.

- **Coarse and/or variable chromatin pattern**
  The cytological evaluation of the chromatin should always be related to the pattern observed in the non-neoplastic counterpart.

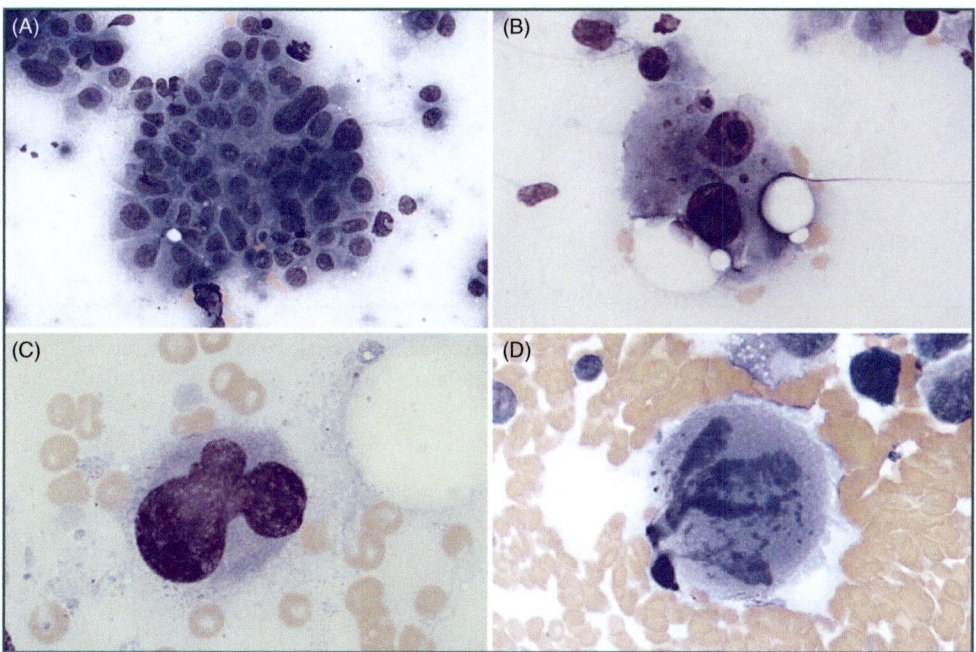

**Fig. 4.1.** Criteria of malignancy. (A) Anisokaryosis and nuclear moulding. (B) Multinucleation, nuclear fragmentation and large prominent nucleoli. (C) Irregular nuclear shape. (D) Atypical mitosis.

- **Mitotic figures**
  The presence of increased numbers of mitoses, especially when atypical (characterized by asymmetrical division), is suggestive of malignancy. Certain cell types (e.g. lymphoid cells, macrophages) may show some degree of mitotic activity in absence of neoplasia.
- **Thickened or irregular nuclear membrane and nuclear blebbing/fragmentation**

## 4.3 Cytoplasmic Criteria

- **Increased cytoplasmic basophilia**
  This should be compared with the normal cell counterpart. Increased basophilia indicates sustained RNA activity, typical of metabolically active cells.
- **Abnormal vacuolation and granulation**

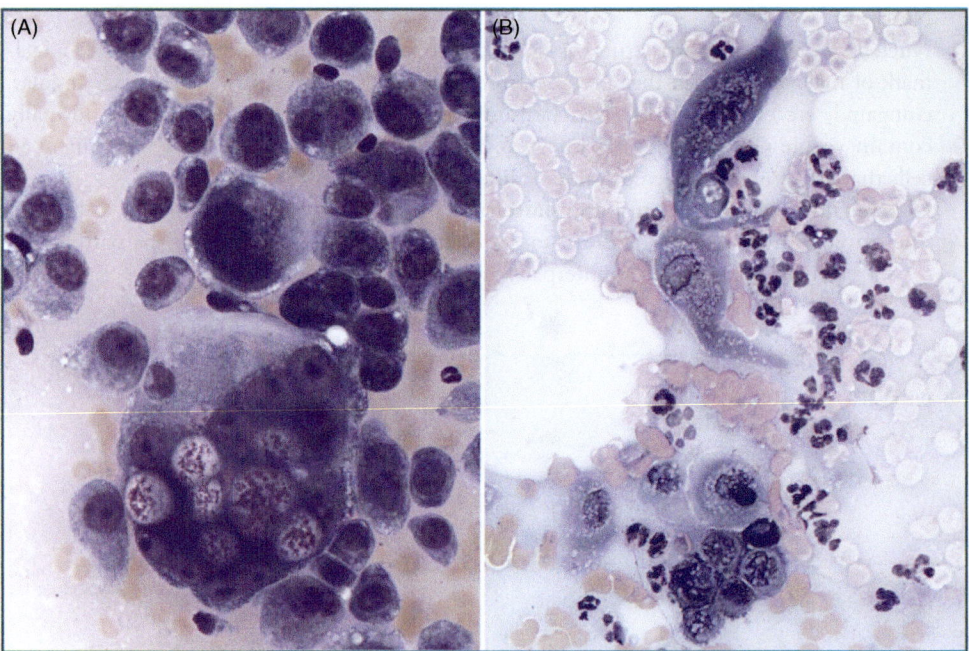

**Fig. 4.2.** Criteria of malignancy. (A) Atypical cytoplasmic vacuolations and reduced cell adhesion (canine urothelial carcinoma). (B) Atypical perinuclear cytoplasmic vacuolation (canine squamous cell carcinoma).

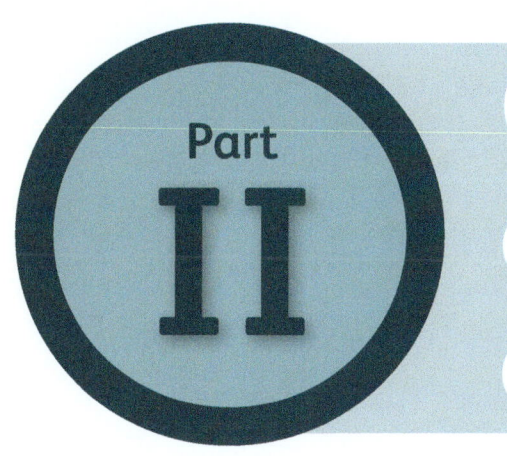

# Part II

# Cytology of Skin and Subcutis

# 5 Skin and Subcutis Anatomy

## 5.1 Main Components of the Skin and Subcutis

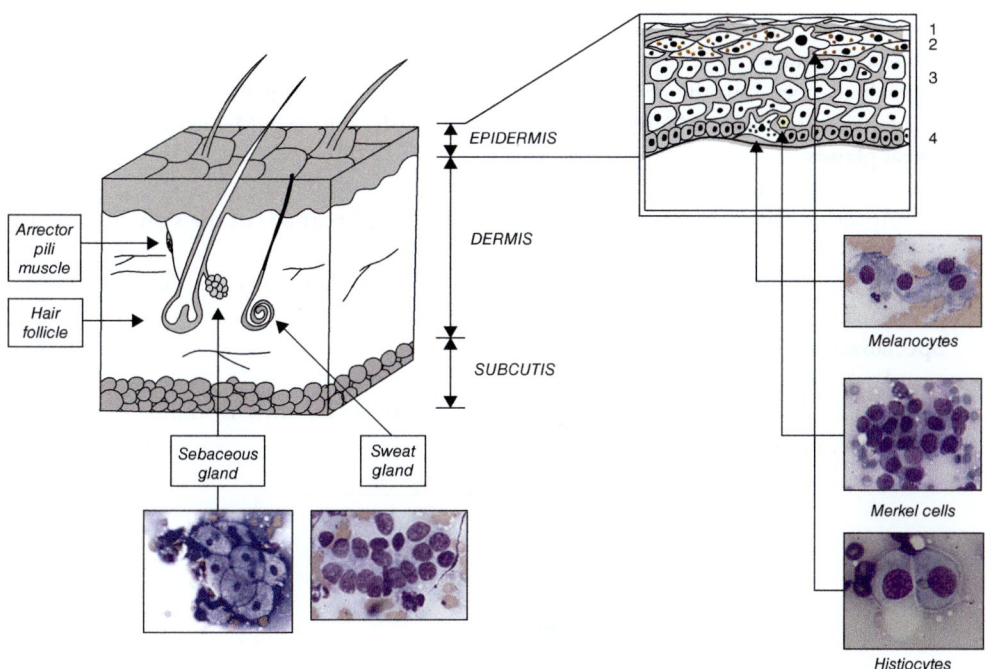

**Fig. 5.1.** Anatomy of the skin. (1) Stratum corneum; (2) Stratum granulosum; (3) Stratum spinosum; (4) Stratum basale.

## Epidermis

The epidermis is mostly composed of keratinocytes. It also contains melanocytes, Langerhans cells (histiocytes) and pressure-sensing Merkel cells. It is formed of four layers:

- Stratum corneum
- Stratum granulosum
- Stratum spinosum
- Stratum basale

## Dermis

The dermis contains collagen, elastic fibres, blood vessels, sensory structures and fibroblasts. It can be subdivided into:

- **Superficial dermis**
  It supports the upper portion of the hair follicles and the sebaceous glands.
- **Deep dermis**
  It contains the lower part of the hair follicle and the apocrine (sweat) glands.

## Subcutis

The subcutis contains adipose tissue, collagenous and elastic fibres and blood vessels. It attaches the dermis to the underlying muscle layer or bone.

## Adnexa

There are different types of adnexa:

- **Sebaceous glands**
  Their ducts open into the hair follicle except for the sebaceous glands located at the mucocutaneous junctions, which open on the surface of the skin (e.g. Meibomian glands).
- **Sweat glands**
  These are of two main types:
  - Apocrine glands are scattered throughout the haired portions of the skin. Their duct opens on the superficial portion of the hair follicle.
  - Eccrine glands are mostly located in the paw pads in dogs and cats. Their duct opens directly on the surface of the epidermis.
- **Specialized structures**
  - Anal sacs are composed of:
    - Sac wall and apocrine cells in dogs. Ducts and sacs are lined by stratified squamous epithelium.

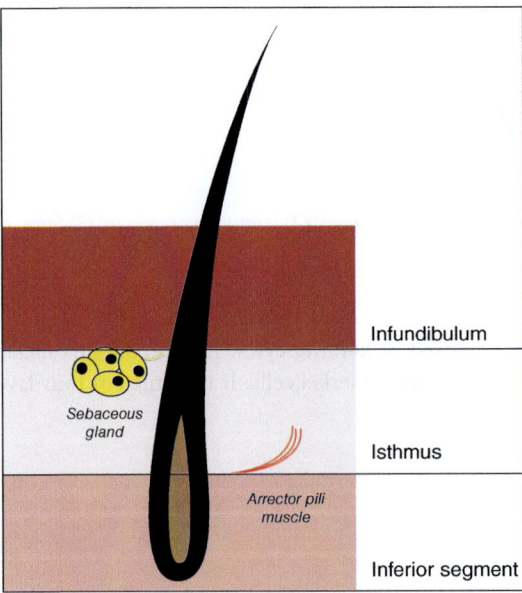

**Fig. 5.2.** Sections of a hair follicle.

- Sac wall, apocrine and sebaceous cells in cats. Ducts and sacs are lined by stratified squamous epithelium.
    - Perianal gland epithelial cells (also called hepatoid glands) are modified sebaceous epithelial cells. They are mostly found around the anus but also near the prepuce, on the tail, flank and groin.
- **Hair follicles**
  Hair follicles consist of an invagination of the epidermis into the dermis. They are responsible for the formation of the hair, which is a modified keratinized structure. They are composed of the following parts:
    - Infundibulum: superficial portion, from the epidermis to the opening of the sebaceous duct.
    - Isthmus: intermediate portion, from the opening of the sebaceous duct to the insertion of the arrector pili muscle.
    - Inferior segment: deep portion from the insertion of the arrector pili muscle to the base of the follicle.

## 5.2 Main Cell Types Observed on Cytology

Different structures and types of epithelial and mesenchymal cells can be seen upon aspiration of cutaneous and subcutaneous lesions.

### Epithelial elements
- Anucleated squamous epithelial cells (keratinocytes) and keratinized material:
    - Polygonal keratinocytes: from the infundibulum of the hair follicle.
    - Liquid keratin material: from the infundibulum of the hair follicle.
    - Amorphous keratinous material: from the isthmus of the hair follicle.
    - Ghost cells: from the inferior segment of the hair follicle.

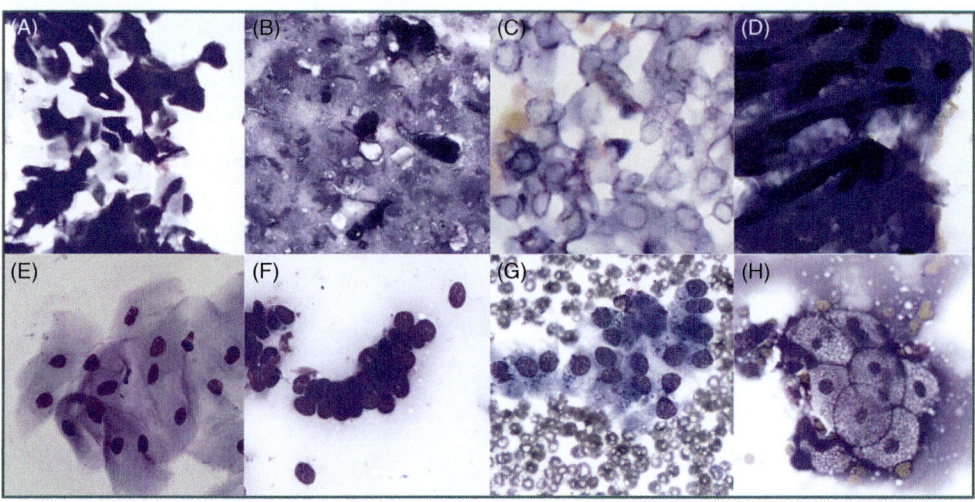

**Fig. 5.3.** Epithelial elements observed in skin cytology. (A) Polygonal keratinocytes. (B) Liquid keratin material. (C) Ghost cells. (D) Hair shafts. (E) Nucleated squamous epithelial cells (keratinocytes). (F) Cuboidal epithelial cells (basaloid epithelial cells). (G) Columnar epithelial cells. (H) Sebocytes.

- Hair shafts.
- Nucleated squamous epithelial cells (keratinocytes): from the epidermis and follicle.
- Cuboidal epithelial cells (basaloid epithelial cells): from the epidermis, follicles, apocrine glands and reserve epithelial cells of the sebaceous and perianal glands.
- Columnar epithelial cells: from the sweat glands.
- Sebocytes: from the sebaceous glands.

## Mesenchymal elements

- Fibroblasts: from the stromal tissue of dermis and subcutis.
- Melanocytes.
- Fragments of skeletal muscle.
- Capillaries.
- Adipocytes: from the subcutaneous tissue.

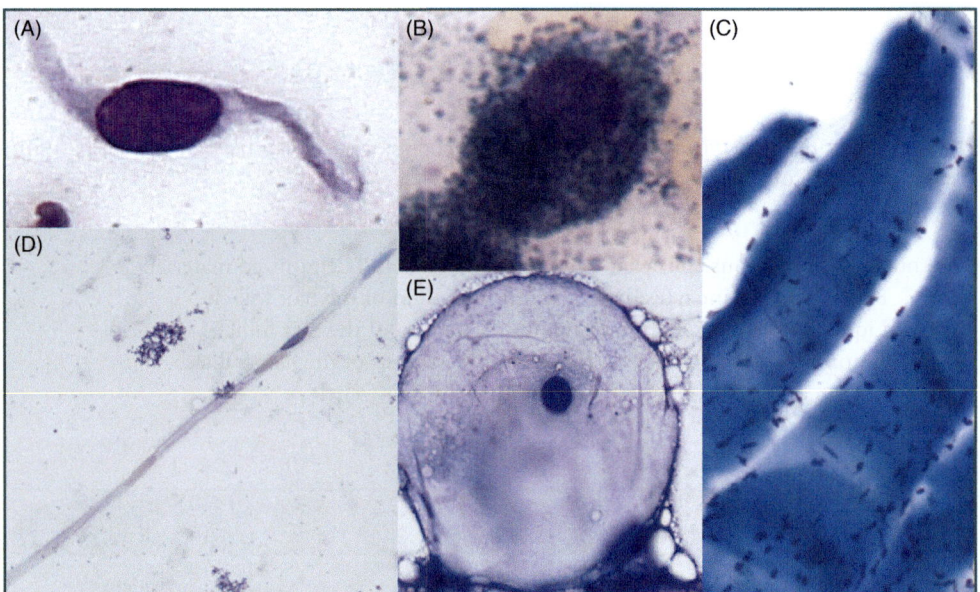

**Fig. 5.4.** Mesenchymal elements observed in skin cytology. (A) Fibroblasts. (B) Melanocytes. (C) Fragments of skeletal muscle. (D) Capillaries. (E) Adipocytes.

# 6  Inflammatory Lesions

Inflammation is classified on cytology based on the predominant cell type involved. It is subdivided into the following categories:

- Neutrophilic
- Macrophagic
- Eosinophilic
- Lymphocytic
- Mixed (in the absence of a prevalent cell type)

The recognition of the inflammatory pattern helps the pathologist to restrict the list of differential diagnoses and sometimes also to identify a potential aetiology. Inflammation can be sterile or associated with an infectious disease. However, the absence of microorganisms on cytology does not rule out an infectious cause, and further testing with a higher sensitivity (e.g. bacterial culture, polymerase chain reaction (PCR)) may be required.

Inflammation may be the sole pathologic process causing the formation of the cutaneous lesion or it may be associated with hyperplastic, dysplastic and neoplastic processes.

The algorithm in Fig. 6.1 shows a correct approach to cutaneous inflammatory lesions.

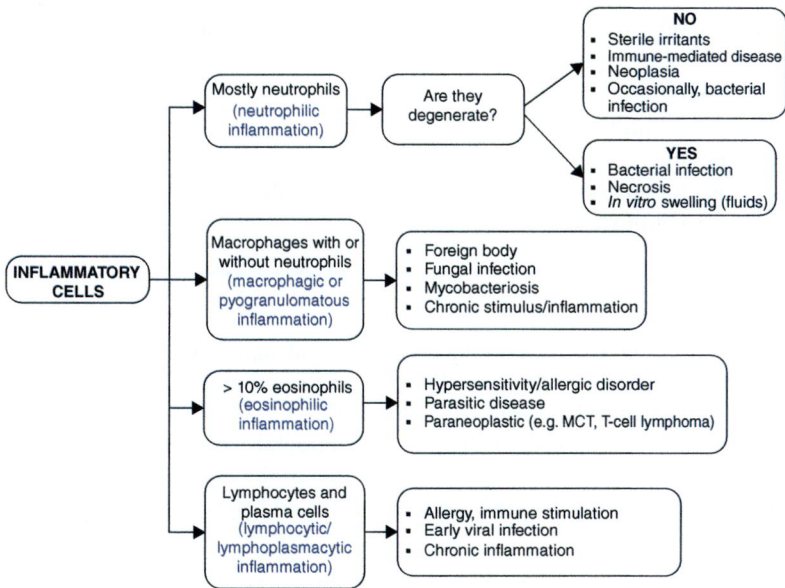

**Fig. 6.1.** Schematic approach to the cytology of inflammatory lesions.

# 6.1 Neutrophilic Inflammation

## General information

- Neutrophils are involved in the innate cell-mediated immunity. One of their key functions is to engulf and neutralize infectious agents (mostly bacteria).

## Cytological features

- Neutrophilic inflammation is diagnosed when the sample contains a vast predominance of neutrophils. Purulent inflammation is sometimes used as a synonym.
- Neutrophils may present in different forms:
  - **Non-degenerate neutrophils**
    Similar to those observed in the circulatory stream. They have segmented, densely stained nuclei with clumped chromatin. Their presence is primarily suggestive of a sterile inflammatory process; however, infection may still be present.
  - **Degenerate neutrophils**
    - Karyolytic neutrophils: characterized by a pale, swollen nucleus with coarse and pale chromatin; typical nuclear segmentation and cell borders may be partially lost. These changes are the result of endotoxins released by the infectious agents that damage the cellular and nuclear membranes, allowing water influx and swelling of cellular components. They are often associated with bacterial and fungal infections. Degenerate neutrophils may also be found in association with severe necrosis.
    - Pyknotic neutrophils: the nucleus loses the typical segmentations and becomes rounder, smaller and denser (apoptosis). This is usually a feature of age-related cell death.
    - Karyorrhectic neutrophils: pyknotic neutrophils following the fragmentation of the nucleus into small fragments.
- Neutrophils may be associated with other cell types, in particular macrophages. In those cases, the inflammation is often referred to as mixed or pyogranulomatous.

## Causes

- Infectious agents (mostly bacteria).
- Trauma/irritation.
- Tissue necrosis (often associated with underlying, rapidly growing neoplasia).
- Immune-mediated process.

---

**Pearls and Pitfalls**
- Care must be taken when diagnosing neutrophilic inflammation in a cytological sample with a significant degree of haemodilution, as the neutrophils could be blood derived, especially if the animal has peripheral neutrophilia.
- On cytology, the diagnosis can be limited to 'neutrophilic inflammation'. In absence of the architecture of the tissue, the exact localization of the inflammatory process cannot be determined and the exact characterization of the underlying pathophysiology cannot always be determined.

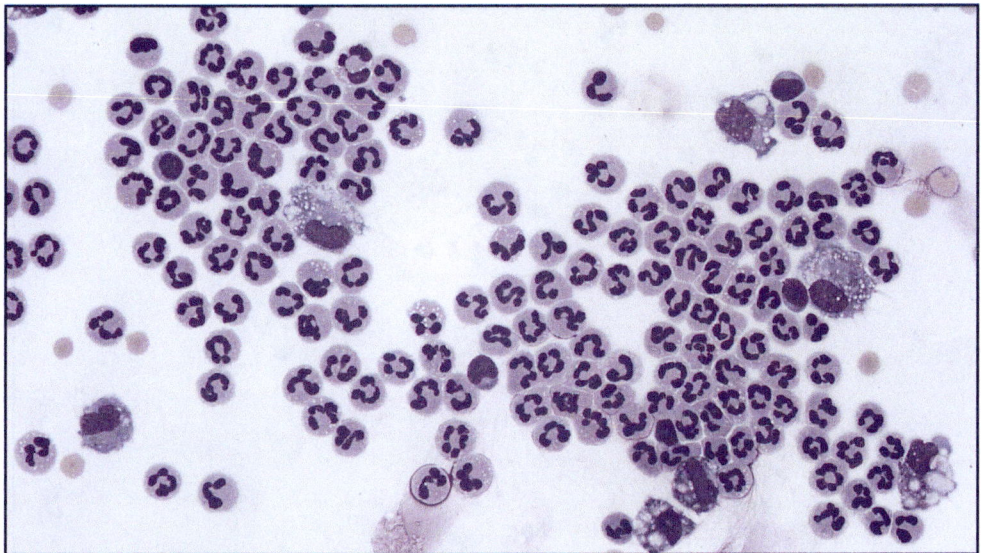

**Fig. 6.2.** Dog. Non-degenerate neutrophils. Wright-Giemsa.

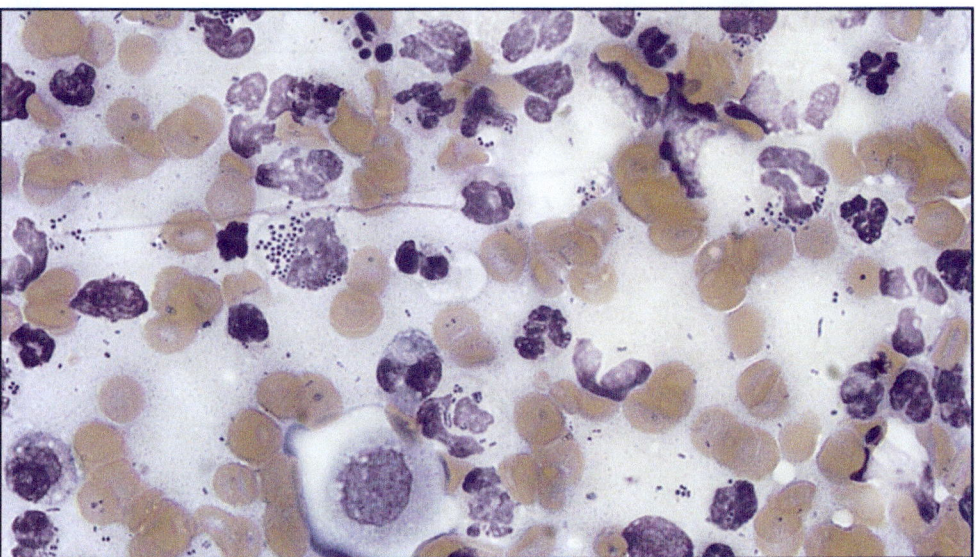

**Fig. 6.3.** Dog. Degenerate neutrophils displaying moderate to marked karyolysis. They occasionally contain phagocytosed bacteria. Wright-Giemsa.

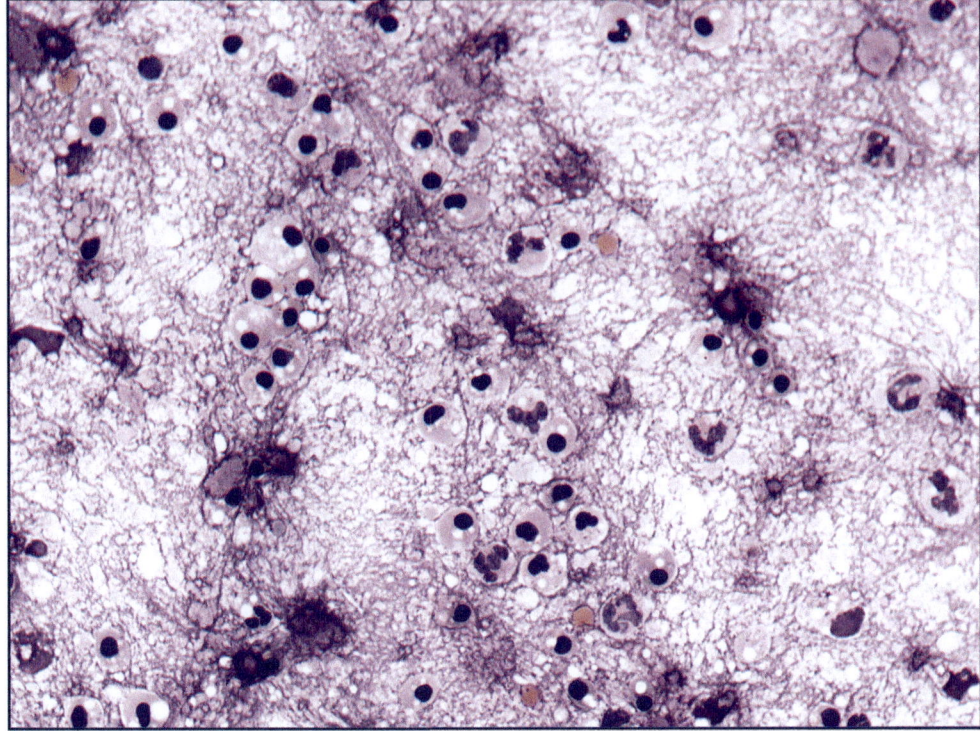

**Fig. 6.4.** Dog. Pyknotic neutrophils. Wright-Giemsa.

# 6.2 Macrophagic Inflammation

## General information

- Macrophages are large mononuclear cells involved in the innate cell-mediated immunity. They originate from circulating monocytes, which migrate into tissues through the endothelium.
- Macrophages are commonly seen in established or chronic inflammatory processes.

## Cytological features

- Macrophagic inflammation is diagnosed when the sample contains a vast predominance of macrophages and is also known as *granulomatous*.
- Macrophagic inflammation may be associated with other inflammatory cells, including neutrophils, lymphocytes and plasma cells. When admixed with neutrophils, the inflammation is referred to as *pyogranulomatous*.
- Other cell types, including epithelioid macrophages, multinucleated giant cells and reactive fibroblasts, may also be present.
    - Epithelioid macrophages: mononuclear cells, often arranged in cohesive groups, with large amounts of uniformly basophilic cytoplasm, overall resembling epithelial cells.
    - Multinucleated giant cells: result of the fusion of multiple epithelioid macrophages. They have a large cytoplasm and contain multiple small nuclei arranged either haphazardly (foreign-body-type giant cells) or peripherally (Langhans-type giant cells).
- Macrophages often display phagocytosis. In haemorrhagic events, they may contain red blood cells (erythrophagocytosis), haemosiderin (haemosiderophages) and/or haematoidin crystals. They can also engulf cellular debris, leucocytes (leucophagia) and/or infectious agents.
- Specific types of macrophagic inflammation (e.g. panniculitis, foreign body/injection reaction) will be discussed in specific chapters.

## Causes

- Selected infectious agents (e.g. *Mycobacterium* spp., *Leishmania* spp., fungi, feline infectious peritonitis (FIP) infection).
- Endogenous or exogenous foreign body reaction.
- Chronic irritation.

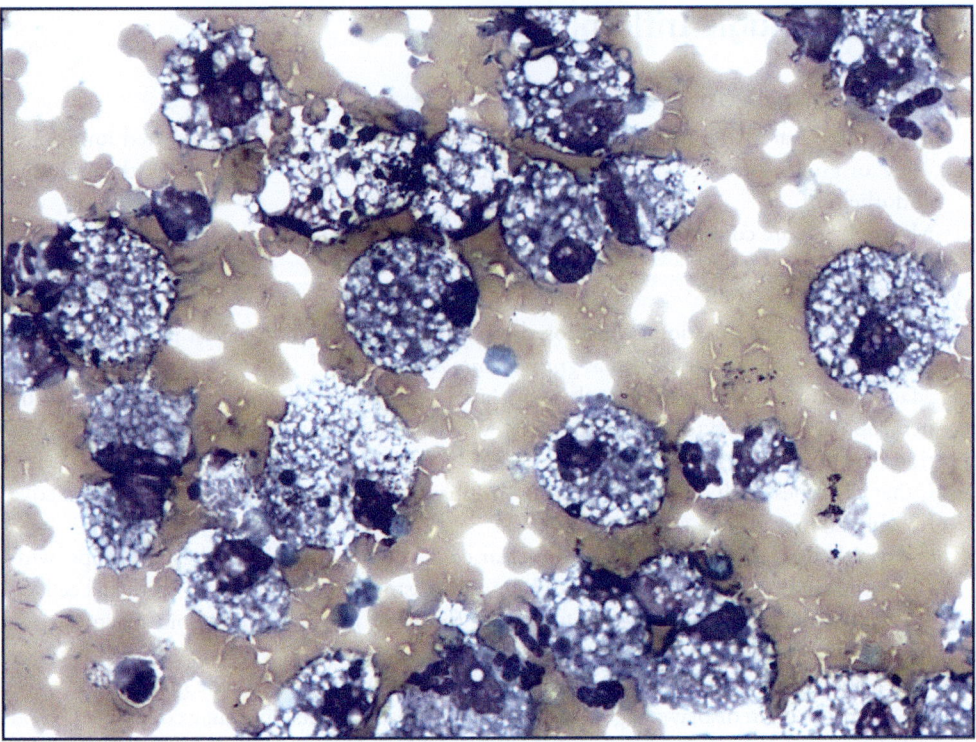

**Fig. 6.5.** Dog. Activated macrophages with signs of phagocytosis in a haemodiluted background. Wright-Giemsa.

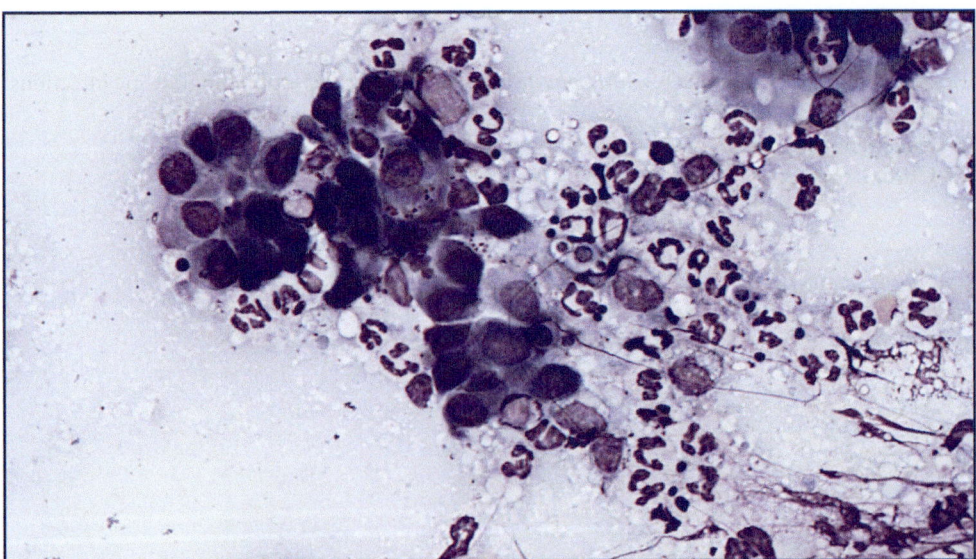

**Fig. 6.6.** Dog. Small cluster of epitheliod macrophages. Fungal pyogranulomatous inflammation. Wright-Giemsa.

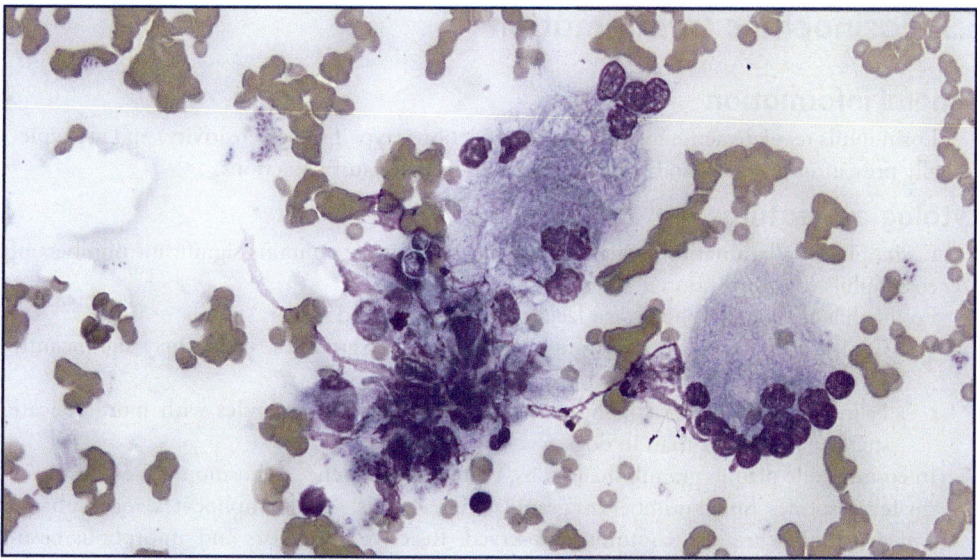

**Fig. 6.7.** Dog. Fungal granulomatous inflammation The multinucleated cell on the right side of the photomicrograph is a Langhans-type giant cell. Nuclei are arranged at the periphery of the cell (horseshoe arrangement). Wright-Giemsa.

## 6.3 Eosinophilic Inflammation

### General information

- Eosinophils regulate acute hypersensitivity reactions (type I hypersensitivity) and are typically present in allergen- and parasite-mediated inflammatory reactions.

### Cytological features

- Eosinophilic inflammation is diagnosed when the sample contains significant numbers of eosinophils (by convention > 10%).
- Eosinophils are polymorphonuclear leucocytes with lobulated nuclei.
  - Canine eosinophils contain round orange to pink granules, which may significantly vary in size and colour.
  - Feline eosinophils contain numerous small rod-shaped granules with more delicate staining properties than in dogs.
- In eosinophilic plaque/granuloma lesions, there is a prevalence of eosinophils, especially in the feline species. Small numbers of granulated mast cells, small lymphocytes, macrophages and neutrophils are also commonly observed. Reactive fibroblasts and amorphous basophilic material may be present as a result of collagenolysis.
- In most of the eosinophilic inflammations caused by hypersensitivity, such as insect/flea-bite reaction, inflammatory cells are often mixed. Eosinophils, small lymphocytes, granulated mast cells, neutrophils and macrophages are present in variable proportions.

### Causes

- Insect-bite reaction.
- Eosinophilic granuloma complex (EGC).
- Immune-mediated process.
- Parasitic or fungal infection.
- Paraneoplastic inflammation (e.g. mast cell tumour, T-cell lymphoma).

---

**Pearls and Pitfalls**

Charcot-Leyden crystals are large eosinophilic structures that result from the coalescence of eosinophil granules into large crystals. They can occur in any condition that causes eosinophils to accumulate.

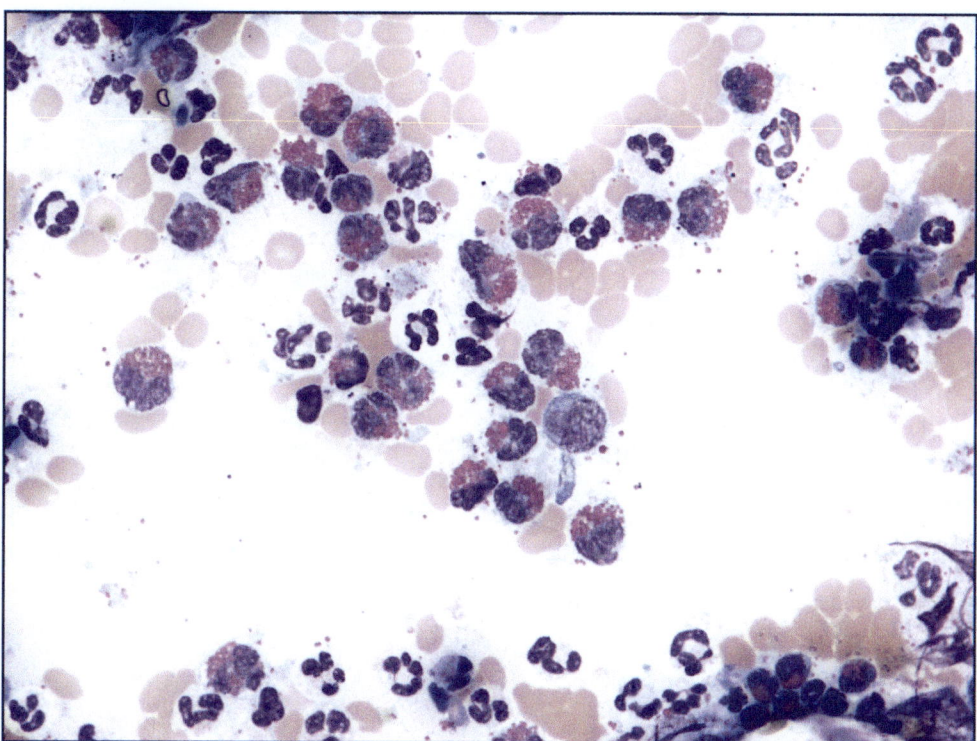

**Fig. 6.8.** Dog. Eosinophilic inflammation. Eosinophilic granules are round. Wright-Giemsa.

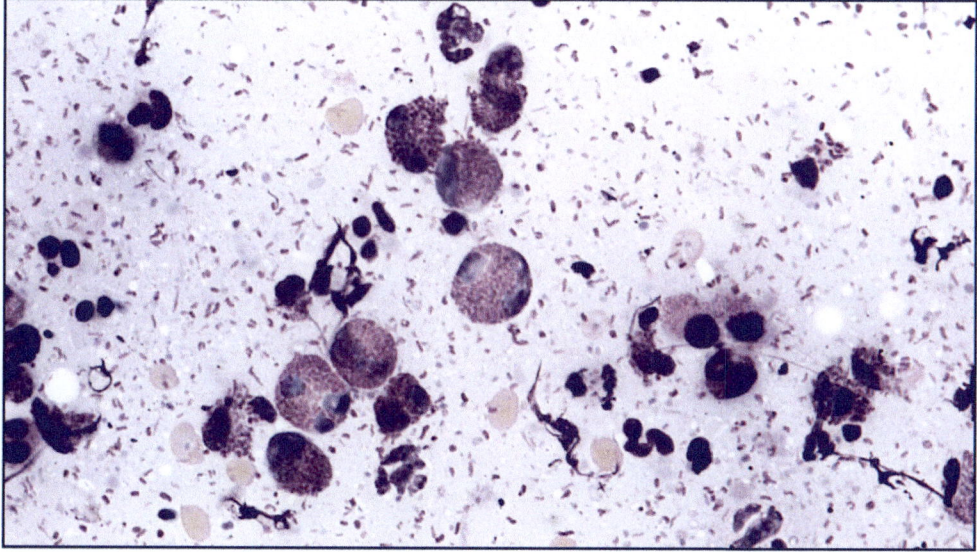

**Fig. 6.9.** Cat. Eosinophilic inflammation. Eosinophilic granules are rod shaped and often seen in the background. Wright-Giemsa.

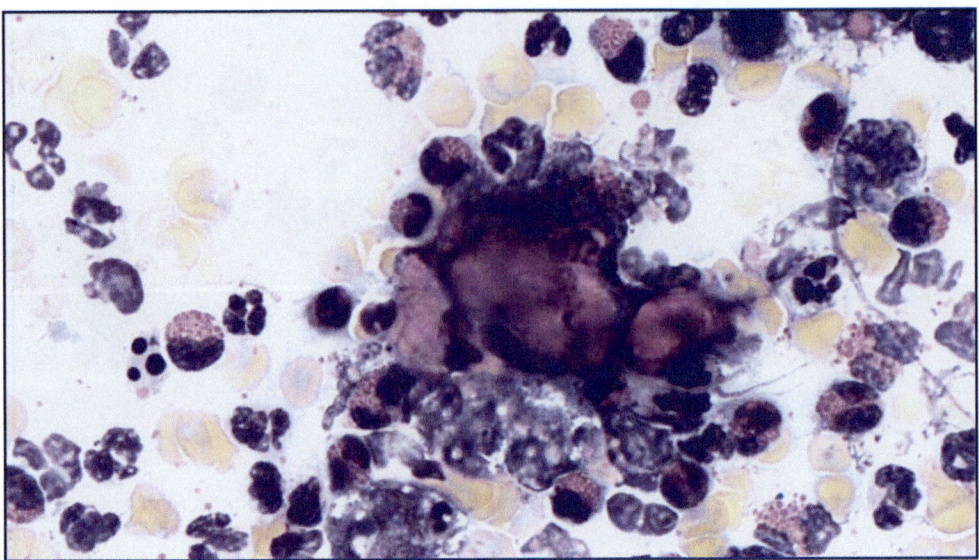

**Fig. 6.10.** Dog. Charcot-Leyden crystal. Wright Giemsa.

# 6.4 Lymphocytic Inflammation

## General information
- Lymphocytes participate in both the humoral and cell-mediated adaptive immune response. They are also involved in type IV (delayed) hypersensitivity reactions.
- They are commonly seen in established or chronic inflammatory processes.

## Cytological features
- Lymphocytic inflammation is diagnosed when the sample contains a vast majority of lymphocytes.
- This type of inflammation is often characterized by a mixed population of lymphoid cells, predominantly small lymphocytes. Low numbers of intermediate and/or large lymphoid cells may also be noted.
- Macrophages and plasma cells can also accompany small lymphocytes in chronic inflammatory processes. When significant numbers of plasma cells are present, the term lymphoplasmacytic inflammation can be used instead.

## Causes
- Non-specific chronic inflammation.
- Vaccine reaction.
- Regressing histiocytoma.
- Insect-bite reaction.
- Viral infection.

---

**Differential diagnoses**
- Cutaneous lymphoma
- Regressing histiocytoma (late stages)

---

**Pearls and Pitfalls**
- Reactive lymphoid follicles may form in the dermis in association with chronic inflammation/stimulation. Aspiration can yield a mixed population of lymphoid cells and lymphoglandular bodies (cytoplasmic fragments).
- In the presence of a main population of small lymphocytes, differentiation between lymphocytic inflammation and small cell lymphoma may not be possible on cytology alone, and it may require additional tests for definitive diagnosis. These include histopathology, immunophenotyping techniques, and/or clonality testing (PARR). When intermediate and/or large lymphoid cells prevail, the diagnosis of (cutaneous) lymphoma is straightforward.

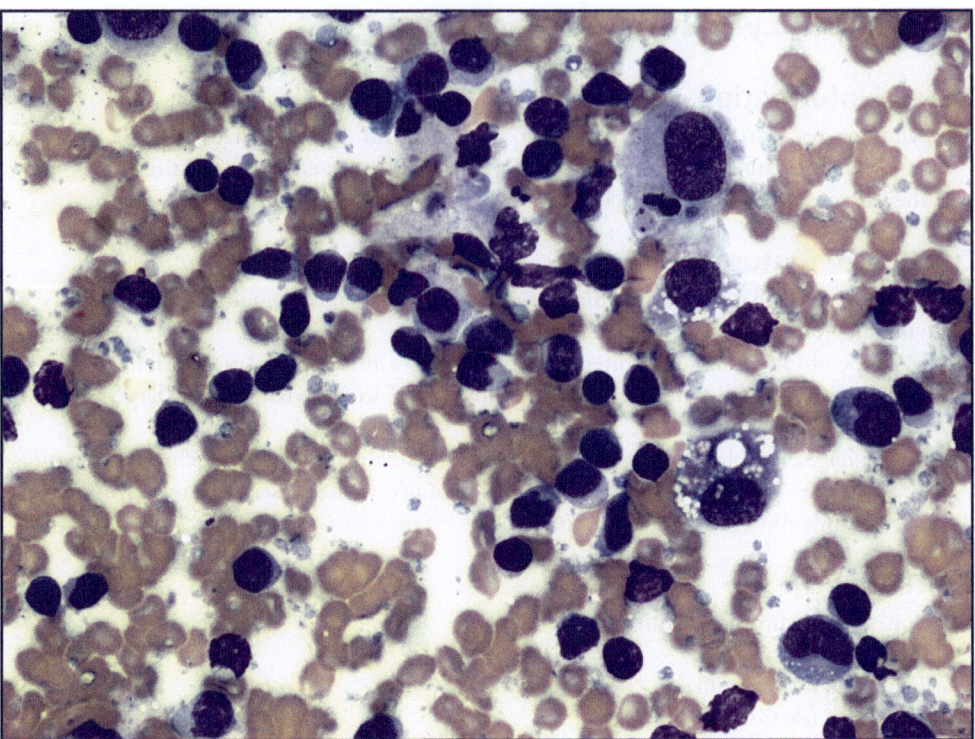

**Fig. 6.11.** Cat. Lymphocytic inflammation. Numerous small lymphocytes are seen in a haemodiluted background. Low numbers of macrophages are also present. Wright-Giemsa.

# 6.5 Inflammation Caused by Infectious Agents

## General information

- Inflammation may be caused by various infectious agents, such as bacteria, fungi, yeasts, algae, protozoa, and/or parasites. Cytological evidence of these organisms, especially when intracellular or associated with the inflammatory cells, is considered proof of infection.
- The absence of microorganisms on the smear does not rule out infection; therefore, additional diagnostic investigations (e.g. culture testing, PCR) may be considered in selected cases.

## Bacterial infections

The presence of intracytoplasmic bacteria (mainly within neutrophils) is the key finding to confirm infection and distinguishing this from sample contamination.

- Bacteria can be differentiated based on their morphology, staining characteristics and sometimes arrangement.
  - Rods or bacilli (e.g. *Proteus* spp., *Pseudomonas* spp., etc.) are elongated and vary in size from small to relatively large, thin or thick. Rod bacteria are usually Gram negative, with the exception of *Corynebacterium* spp., which is Gram positive.
  - Cocci are round (spherical) and can be found in chains (e.g. *Streptococcus* spp.) or groups (e.g. *Staphylococcus* spp.). Most cocci are Gram positive.
  - Filamentous bacteria, e.g. *Nocardia* spp., *Actinomyces* spp.
  - Negatively staining rods: *Mycobacterium* spp.
- Bacteria commonly cause a neutrophilic inflammatory response, often associated with the presence of degenerate forms. The exception to this is *Mycobacterium* spp., which more frequently cause a pyogranulomatous or granulomatous response.

## Fungal, yeasts or algae infections

- Aetiological agents: fungi, yeasts or algae.
- Partial identification can be attempted by morphological examination (e.g. *Cryptococcus* spp., *Malassezia canis* or *M. pachydermatis*), but culture or PCR testing is required for precise characterization.
- They often elicit a neutrophilic and/or macrophagic inflammatory response, with a variable eosinophilic component.
- The hyphae can be found phagocytosed by the macrophages and/or surrounded by the inflammatory cells.

## Protozoal infections

- Aetiological agents; for example:
  - *Leishmania* spp.
  - *Toxoplasma gondii.*
  Protozoa often elicit a mixed but predominantly macrophagic inflammation. Plasma cells may also be seen associated with *Leishmania* infection.

## Parasitic infections

- Aetiological agents; for example:
  - Mites (e.g. *Sarcoptes* spp., *Demodex* spp., *Cheyletiella* spp.)
  - *Dirofilaria repens.*
  Parasites usually trigger a neutrophilic to pyogranulomatous inflammation with a variable eosinophilic component.

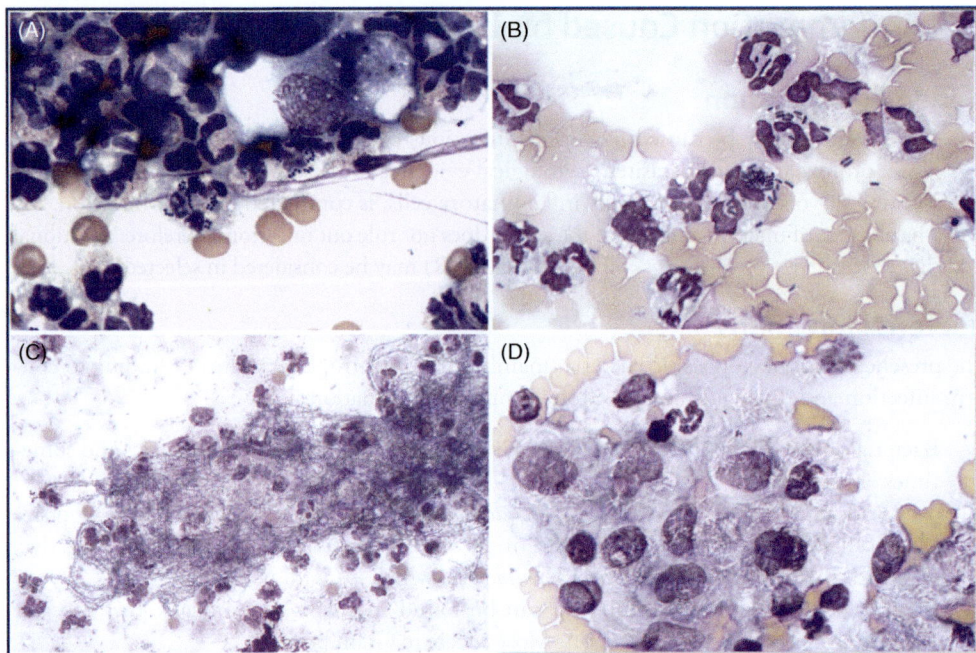

**Fig. 6.12.** Bacteria. (A) Cocci. (B) Rods. (C) *Actinomyces.* (D) *Mycobacteria* spp. Wright-Giemsa.

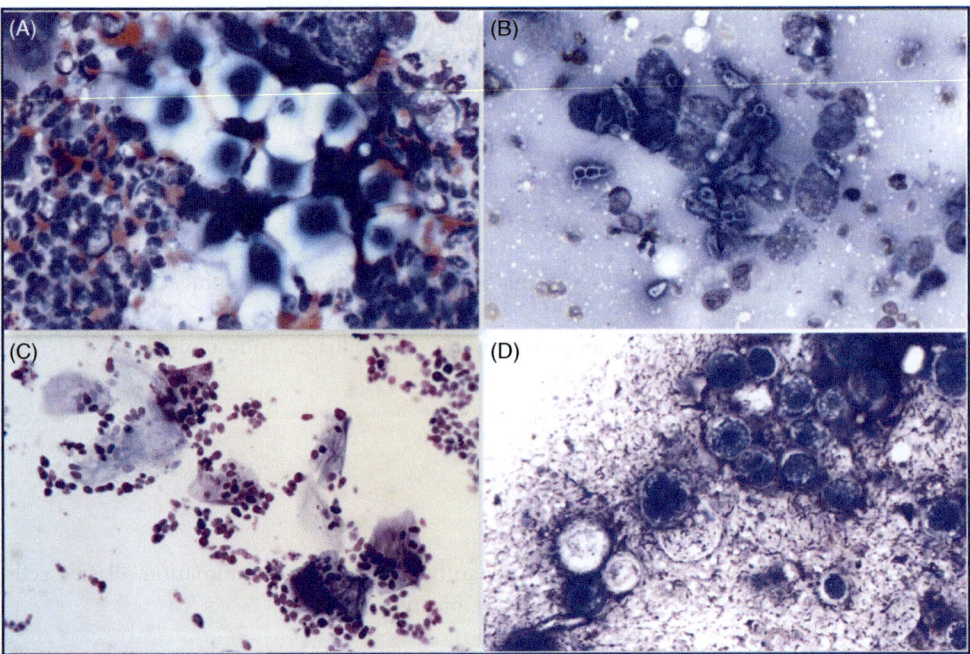

**Fig. 6.13.** Fungi and algae. (A) *Cryptococcus* spp.: multiple round basophilic structures with thick and clear capsules. (B) Pseudohyphae of *Candida albicans*: septated tubular walls with typical constrictions at the positions of septa. They are seen phagocytosed by macrophages and free in the background. (C) *Malassezia* spp.: budding yeasts typically peanut-shaped. (D) Prototheca: variably sized, round to oval structures with a clear cell wall, a small nucleus and a basophilic cytoplasm. Wright-Giemsa.

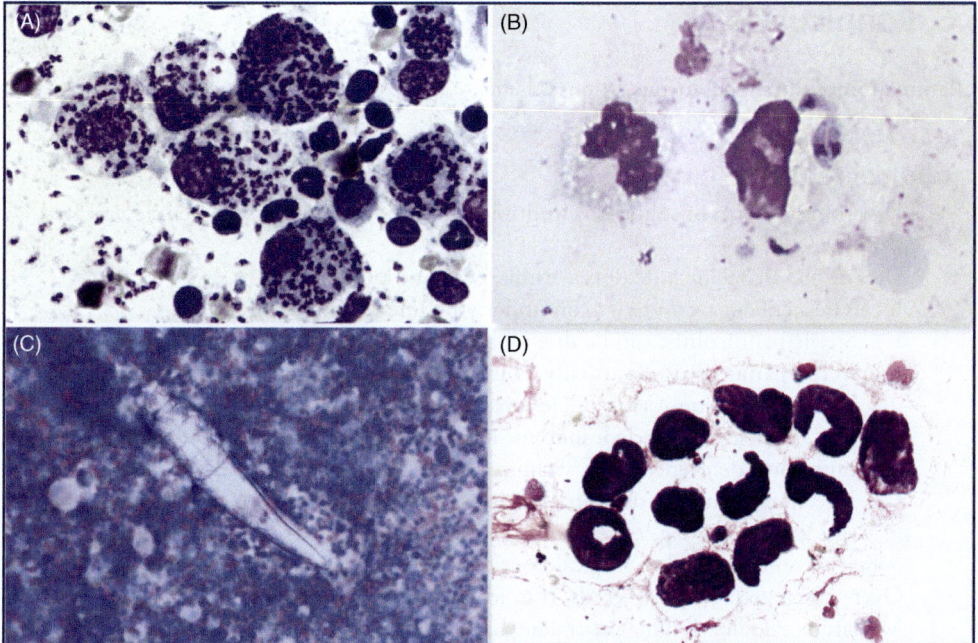

**Fig. 6.14.** Protozoa and parasites. (A) *Leishmania* spp.: numerous amastigotes are seen within macrophages and free in the background. They measure approximately 2–4 µm and are oval with small purple nuclei, small rod-shaped kinetoplasts and clear cytoplasm. (B) *Toxoplasma* spp.: small tachizoites are seen in the centre of the picture. They are banana-shaped with small purple nuclei and tapered clear cytoplasmic tails. Tachizoites usually measure 5–50 µm. (C) *Demodex* spp.: one negatively staining organism is seen admixed with numerous degenerate neutrophils. It has a thin body and four pairs of legs. (D) *Dirofilaria repens*: numerous 'egg cells' containing small larvae. Wright-Giemsa.

## 6.6 Panniculitis

Inflammation of the subcutaneous adipose tissue.

### Clinical features
- Presenting in form of solitary or multiple, firm to fluctuant, raised, well demarcated lesions.
- Sites of prevalence include dorsal trunk, neck and proximal limbs.
- It can be sterile or secondary to an underlying infectious disease.
  - Sterile panniculitis: can be due to a localized or systemic disease. Focal areas of sterile panniculitis are usually caused by trauma, foreign bodies, vaccination/injection reactions. Multiple lesions are often associated with a systemic condition. Possible causes include immune-mediated diseases, drug reactions, pancreatitis, nutritional deficiencies (e.g. vitamin E) and idiopathic disease.
  - Infectious panniculitis: can be caused by bacteria (including *Mycobacterium* spp.), protozoa (e.g. *Leishmania* spp.) and fungi.
- Solitary lesions respond to surgical excision and are associated with good prognosis.
- Over-represented canine breeds (for idiopathic sterile panniculitis): Dachshund, Miniature Poodle, Collie, Australian Shepherd, Brittany, Dalmatian, Pomeranian and Chihuahua.

### Cytological features
- Cellularity is variable, often adequate.
- Background: characterized by numerous variable-sized, clear fat droplets. Often pale basophilic (proteinaceous), it might be variably haemodiluted.
- Amorphous foreign material (e.g. mineral salts) may be seen in panniculitis secondary to drug injections.
- The type of inflammation depends on the underlying cause and duration of the process. Macrophages are most frequently seen. They typically contain numerous small, clear punctate vacuoles of lipids, and occasionally small amorphous phagosomes. Multinucleated cells can be present.
- Neutrophils are seen in acute processes and in association with bacterial infection.
- Small lymphocytes may be numerous, especially in lesions associated with vaccine/injection reaction.
- Reactive fibroblasts are frequently present intermingled with the inflammatory cells.
- Variable numbers of mature adipocytes, intact or necrotic, can be present.

### Differential diagnoses
- Xanthoma (rare)
- Liposarcoma

**Pearls and Pitfalls**

- Idiopathic sterile nodular panniculitis is a descriptive term used to indicate a sterile inflammatory disease of the subcutaneous fat for which the triggering aetiology is unknown. It presents as multiple subcutaneous nodules, often ulcerated, fistulated and draining a lipid material mixed with blood. The trunk is the most commonly affected anatomical area. This form is often associated with systemic clinical signs, such as fever, anorexia and malaise. The Dachshund breed is considered at increased risk.

- Juvenile sterile granulomatous dermatitis and lymphadenitis (also called puppy strangles or juvenile cellulitis, as the inflammation often extends to the subcutis) is a disease of unknown origin affecting young dogs (puppies). Clinically, it is characterized by swelling and exudation of the skin of ears, eyelids, lips, nose and mucucutaneous junctions. Submandibular lymph nodes may be enlarged and systemic clinical signs of malaise are common. Cocker Spaniel, Dachshund and Gordon Setter dogs seem more frequently represented. A pyogranulomatous process with prevalence of neutrophils and macrophages is observed on cytology.

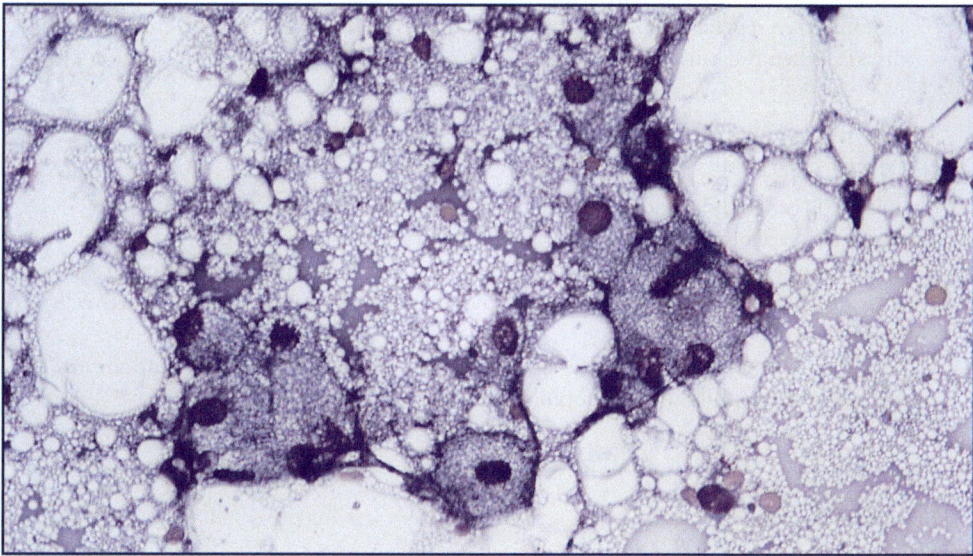

**Fig. 6.15.** Dog. Panniculitis secondary to trauma. The background is proteinaceous and contains numerous punctate fat droplets. Multiple macrophages are seen. They have abundant cytoplasm containing high numbers of lipid vacuoles. Wright-Giemsa.

# Further reading

Countreary, C.L., Outerbridge, C.A., Affolter, V., Kass, P.H. and White, S.D. (2015) Canine sterile nodular panniculitis: a retrospective study of 39 dogs. *Veterinary Dermatology* 26, 451–458.

O'Kell, A.L., Inteeworn, N., Diaz, S.F., Saunders, G.K. and Panciera, D.L. (2010) Canine sterile nodular panniculitis: a retrospective study of 14 cases. *Journal of Veterinary Internal Medicine* 24, 278–284.

## 6.7 Xanthoma

Deposition in the dermis of cholesterol, triglyceride and/or phospholipids causing a granulomatous inflammation.

### Clinical features

- Rare in cats and very rare in dogs.
- It is the result of abnormal plasma concentrations of cholesterol, triglycerides or lipoproteins, which may deposit into tissues, including skin.
- It may be secondary to high-fat diet feeding, diabetes mellitus or idiopathic hyperlipidaemia. In the cat, it has also been associated with secondary hyperlipidaemia due to glucocorticoid or progesterone therapy. Trauma may play a role in the formation of xanthoma.
- It presents as multiple pale yellow to white papules, plaques or nodules, often oozing material upon aspiration.
- In cats, it occurs more often in the preauricular and periorbital region and, to a lesser extent, elsewhere on the head, pinnae, neck, legs and bony prominences. Similar locations and ventrum are seen in dogs.
- Lesions may regress spontaneously with successful management of the primary disease, when present.

### Cytological features

- Cellularity is generally adequate.
- Background: variably haemodiluted. Cholesterol crystals may be seen.
- Variable numbers of macrophages with abundant foamy cytoplasm containing frequent clear distinct vacuoles, compatible with lipid material. Bi- and multinucleated cells are commonly seen.
- Other inflammatory cell types may also be present, in particular small lymphocytes and occasionally neutrophils and eosinophils.

**Differential diagnosis**
Panniculitis

### Pearls and Pitfalls

- Xanthoma and panniculitis cannot be easily differentiated cytologically. The features reported in the table below can be used as a guideline to differentiate these two forms.

|  | Panniculitis | Xanthoma |
|---|---|---|
| Frequency | Relatively frequent | Rare |
| Clinical manifestation | Subcutaneous nodules, often solitary or occasionally multiple | Multiple pale yellow to white papules, plaques, or nodules |
| Localization in tissue | Subcutis | Dermis |
| Presence of adipocytes on cytology | Often present | Often absent (unless incidental aspiration of the subcutaneous fat occurs) |

- Cytochemical stains may be used to confirm the presence of lipid-laden macrophages. With Oil Red O, lipid material stains bright red.

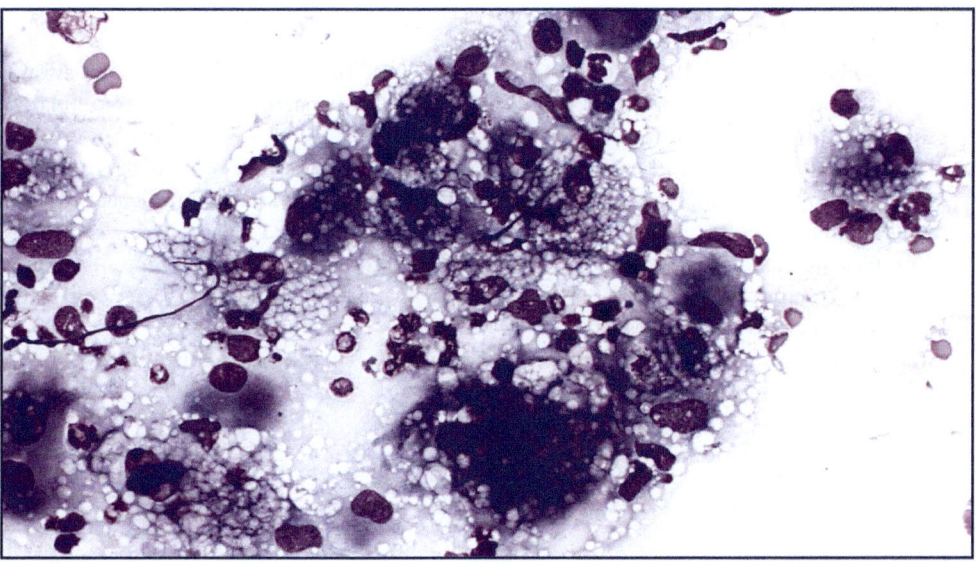

**Fig. 6.16.** Cat. Xanthoma. Activated macrophages are present. They contain numerous punctate clear vacuoles (lipids). Wright-Giemsa. (*Courtesy of Tracy Stokol, Cornell University, USA.*)

## Further reading

Bajajee, K.H., Orandle, M.S., Ratterree, W., Bauer, R.W. and Gaunt, S.D. (2011) Idiopathic solitary cutaneous xanthoma in a dog. *Veterinary Clinical Pathology* 40(1), 95–98.

# 6.8 Injection Site and Foreign Body Reaction

Inflammatory process triggered by injection, most typically vaccinations or other foreign bodies.

## Clinical features

- Caused by either endogenous or exogenous foreign body (FB) material.
  - Endogenous FB material: keratin. This inflammatory process is often observed associated with follicular cysts or cystic follicular tumours. It occurs following the rupture of the cystic wall and exposure of the keratin to the surrounding tissues.
  - Exogenous FB material: vaccine adjuvant, plant material, suture material, surgical swabs or sponges, etc.
- Solitary or multiple nodules in any area of the body. When induced by vaccinations/injections, nodules are most commonly observed in the intrascapular area or hindlimb muscles.
- Spontaneous regression is possible but surgical exploration/excision is often required and carries a good prognosis.

## Cytological features

- Cellularity is variable, often moderate to high.
- Background: variably haemodiluted and proteinaceous. The foreign material is not always found. If present, it may be found in the cytoplasm of the macrophages or extracellularly, surrounded by the inflammatory cells.
- Inflammatory cells are often mixed. Recent or infected processes are often pyogranulomatous and a mixture of macrophages, degenerate neutrophils and variable numbers of eosinophils are found.
- Chronic inflammations are characterized by numerous macrophages alongside small lymphocytes and plasma cells. Both epithelioid macrophages and multinucleated giant inflammatory cells can be present.
- In vaccine/injection-associated reactions, small lymphocytes may be numerous and eosinophils can be found in significant numbers.
- Variable numbers of reactive fibroblasts can be present.
- Tissue necrosis may occur.

### Differential diagnosis

Pyogranulomatous or granulomatous inflammation caused by infectious agents (e.g. fungi, bacteria)

### Pearls and Pitfalls

Occasionally, Langhans cells can be seen in chronic granulomatous inflammations. They represent a variant of the multinucleated giant cells. Their nuclei are typically positioned at the periphery of the cell, in a horseshoe type of arrangement. They can be found in fungal infections, mycobacteriosis or in any other case of granulomatous reaction.

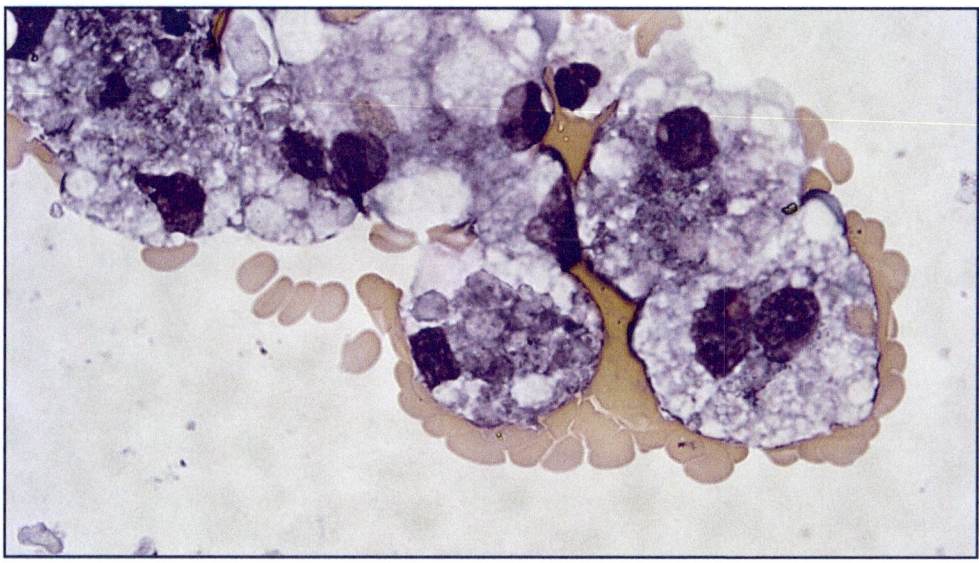

**Fig. 6.17.** Cat. Macrophagic inflammation triggered by previous injection. Activated macrophages contain a pale basophilic refractile amorphous material compatible with the adjuvant present in vaccines. Wright-Giemsa.

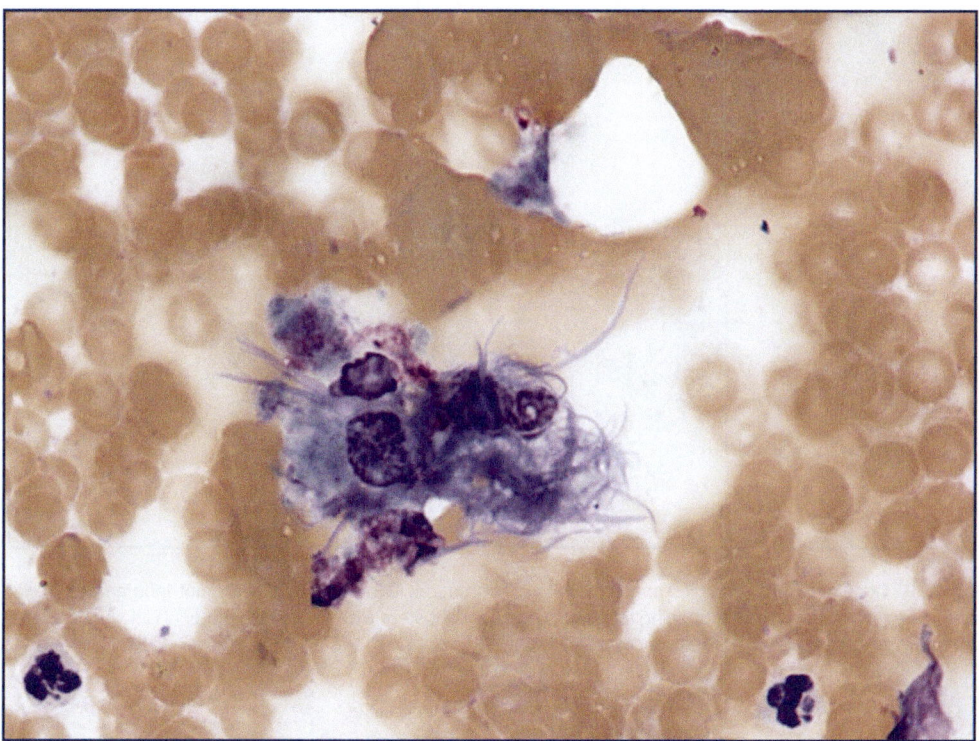

**Fig. 6.18.** Dog. Macrophages containing elongate pale basophilic structures compatible with cotton fibres. Foreign-body reaction secondary to surgical swab. Wright-Giemsa.

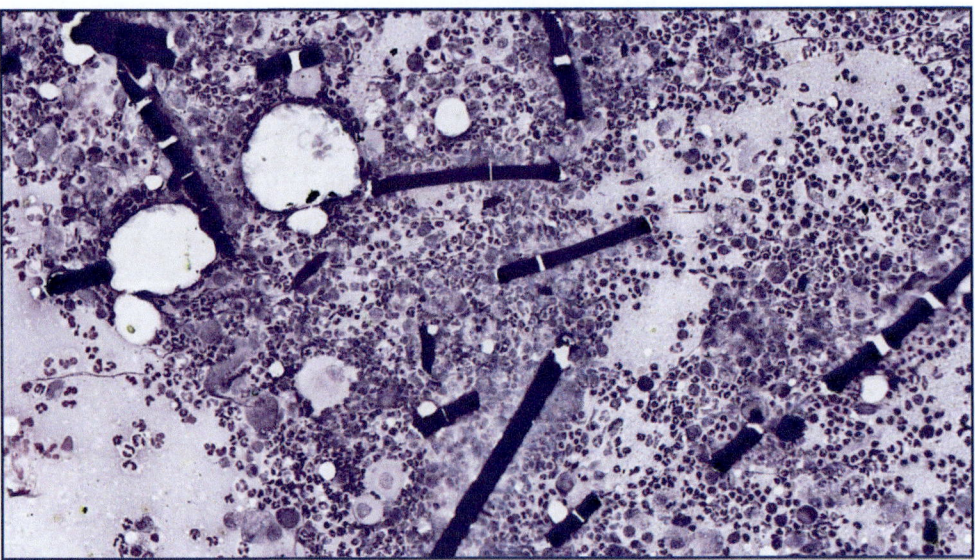

**Fig. 6.19.** Dog. Pyogranulomatous inflammation. Foreign-body reaction caused by suture material following surgery. The suture material appears as regular elongated, deeply basophilic structures with small interruptions. Wright-Giemsa.

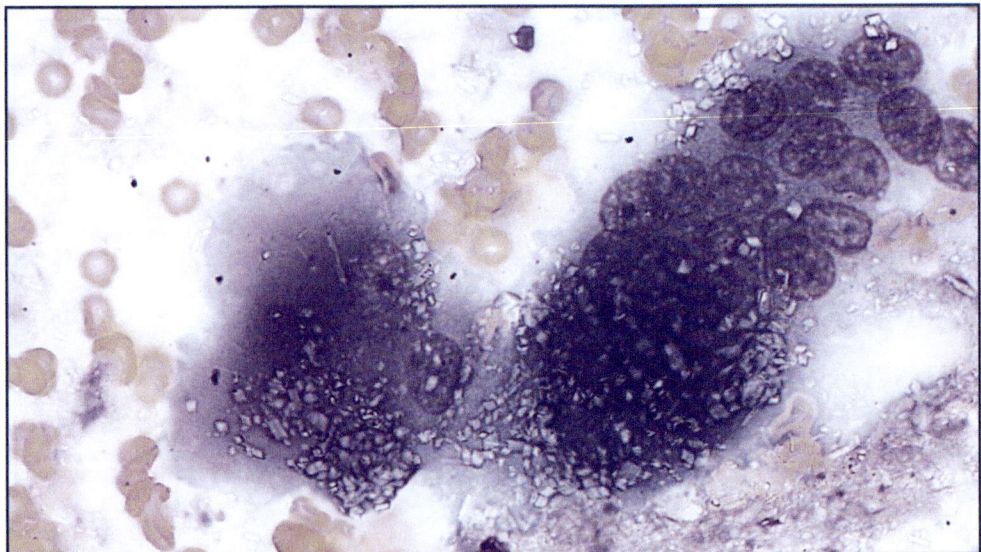

**Fig. 6.20.** Dog. Swelling of a digit. Granulomatous inflammation. Two multinucleated giant inflammatory cells containing numerous negatively staining refractile structures consistent with exogenous material (origin unknown). Similar structures are also seen in the background. Wright-Giemsa.

# 6.9 Pemphigus foliaceus (PF)

Autoimmune blistering process caused by the production of autoantibodies against antigens on the surface of the keratinocytes of the epidermis.

## Clinical features
- Uncommon condition in dogs and cats.
- Average age in dogs is 4 years with two-thirds of subjects developing lesions at or before 5 years of age. Age predilection not reported in cats.
- It presents in the form of pustules or crusts of variable sizes and colours. They are located on the muzzle, planum nasale, pinnae, periorbital area and distal extremities, including paw pads. In dogs, the nose often appears inflamed and depigmented with crusts; trunk, ventral abdomen, scrotum and mucucutaneous junctions can also be involved.
- Causes of pemphigus foliaceus are mostly unknown. Some cases have been linked to chronic skin disease and allergy. In cats, a drug-related PF-like condition has been described after administration of selected antibiotics and methimazole.
- Pemphigus foliaceus is a progressive disease with variable response to treatment.
- Over-represented canine breeds: Bearded Collie, Akita, Chow Chow, Newfoundland, Schipperke, Dobermann, English Springer Spaniel, Shar Pei and Collie.

## Cytological features
- Cellularity is variable, often good.
- Background: variably haemodiluted.
- Variable numbers of acantholytic keratinocytes, characterized by a moderate to abundant amount of basophilic cytoplasm. The cell borders are rounded. Nuclei are round, centrally located, often showing a single prominent nucleolus.
- High numbers of non-degenerate neutrophils are often present. These cells can be found encircling the acantholytic cells.
- Eosinophils are present in about half of the dogs with PF.

**Differential diagnosis**
Bacterial superficial folliculitis

**Pearls and Pitfalls**
- In order to increase the chances of identifying acantolytic cells, impression smears from the inner surface of the crusts are preferred over the exclusive cytological examination of the purulent material. For similar reasons, when incisional biopsies are taken, early lesions (e.g. pustules and vesicopustules) should be included.
- Other less common forms of pemphigus (e.g. pemphigus vulgaris, pemphigus erythematosus) have been reported in the dog and the cat. These are cytologically indistinguishable from pemphigus foliaceus and definitive diagnosis relies on clinical and histopathological findings.
- Acantolytic cells are not pathognomonic for pemphigus and can also be found in association with other types of inflammatory skin diseases and neoplasia.

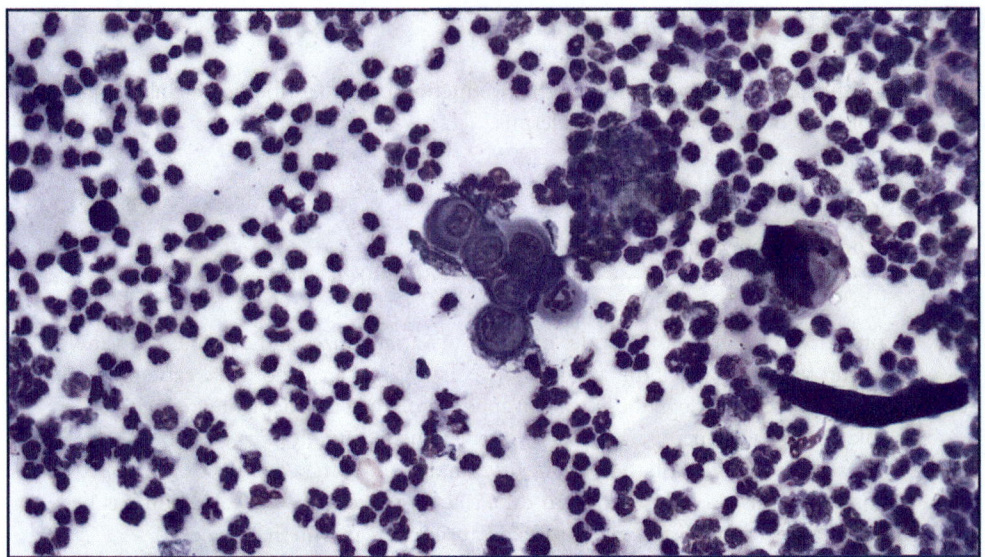

**Fig. 6.21.** Dog. Pemphigus foliaceus. A small group of acantholytic cells is seen in the centre of the photograph. Neutrophilic inflammation. Wright-Giemsa.

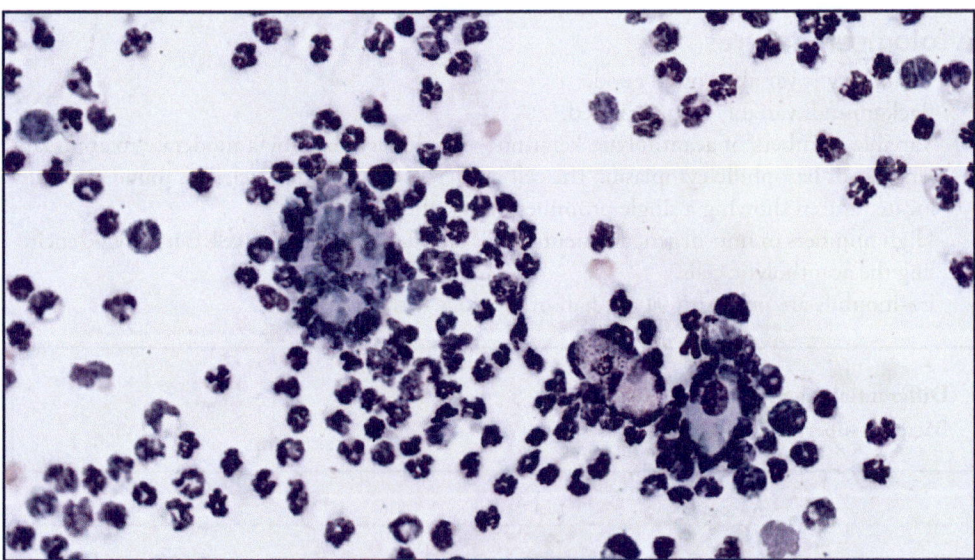

**Fig. 6.22.** Dog. Pemphigus foliaceus. The keratinocytes are surrounded by the inflammatory cells, which are targeting antigens on their surface. Wright-Giemsa.

# 7

# Cysts, Tumour-like Lesions and Response to Tissue Injury

To this category belong all those lesions that may arise in the skin or subcutis and that are not strictly inflammatory or neoplastic. These include follicular or adnexal cysts, developmental anomalies, response to tissue trauma, altered deposition of minerals, necrosis and tumour-like proliferations. Most of these processes can be identified on cytology; however, sometimes definitive diagnosis relies on histopathological examination.

## 7.1 Follicular Cysts

Non-neoplastic, sac-like cavities arising in the hair follicle and lined by stratified squamous epithelium.

### Clinical features
- Relatively common in dogs, less frequent in cats.
- Age: most commonly seen in adult animals.
- They can occur in any location, but most commonly arise on the head and trunk.
- Usually occur as single masses, less frequently as multiple (e.g. German Shepherd Dog and Pekingese). A small pore can occasionally be found on the surface of the lesion. Masses can be ulcerated.
- Usually confined to the dermis. Larger cysts may extend into the subcutaneous adipose tissue.
- They are benign lesions; however, rupture of the cystic wall and exposure of the keratin to the surrounding tissues can elicit an endogenous foreign body reaction characterized by a neutrophilic to pyogranulomatous inflammation.

### Cytological features
- Aspirates usually exfoliate a moderate to large amount of specimen.
- Background: clear or pale basophilic. It may contain cholesterol crystals and hair shafts.
- High numbers of anucleated squamous epithelial cells exfoliate singly or in large groups. Amorphous dense keratin can also be observed.
- Neutrophils, macrophages and/or multinucleated giant inflammatory cells can be seen in inflamed cysts.

### Variants
- Follicular cysts can be classified as *infundibular*, *isthmic*, *matrical* and *hybrid*, based on the type of lining epithelium of the cystic wall. However, this classification does not have any clinical implication and the general term of follicular cyst is most frequently used.

- **Infundibular cyst**

  Usually exfoliates numerous anucleated squamous epithelial cells. These are intact and with well defined margins. They vary from being lightly to moderately basophilic. Occasionally, they may be embedded in a watery basophilic background of keratinic material.

- **Isthmic cyst**

  Aspirates usually contain pale, amorphous and homogeneous keratin.

- **Matrical cyst**

  Characterized by the exfoliation of variable numbers of ghost cells (description of ghost cells can be found in the pilomatricoma section in Chapter 8).

- **Hybrid cyst**

  This type of cyst contains a mixture of the anucleated squames and keratinized material typical of the other cysts described above.

---

**Differential diagnoses**

- Infundibular keratinizing acanthoma (no ghost cells seen)
- Trichoepithelioma
- Pilomatricoma

---

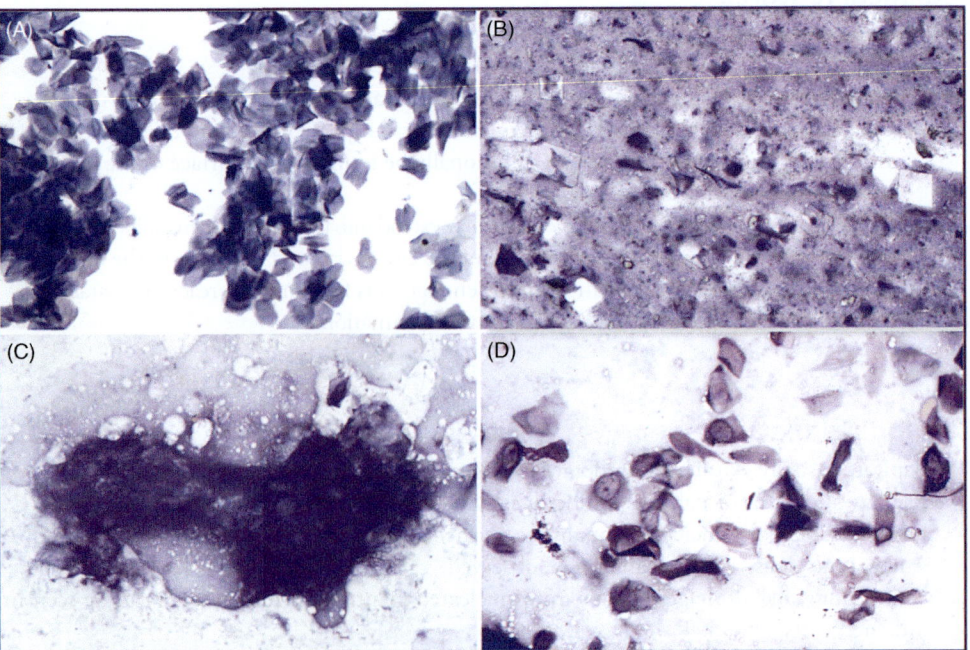

**Fig. 7.1.** Dog. Variants of follicular cyst. (A) Polygonal anucleated squamous epithelial cells suggestive of an infundibular cyst. (B) Liquid keratin with low numbers of lamellar anucleated squamous epithelial cells suggestive of an infundibular cyst. Cholesterol crystals are also observed. (C) Dense and homogeneous keratin suggestive of an isthmic cyst. (D) Ghost cells suggestive of a matrical cyst. Wright-Giemsa.

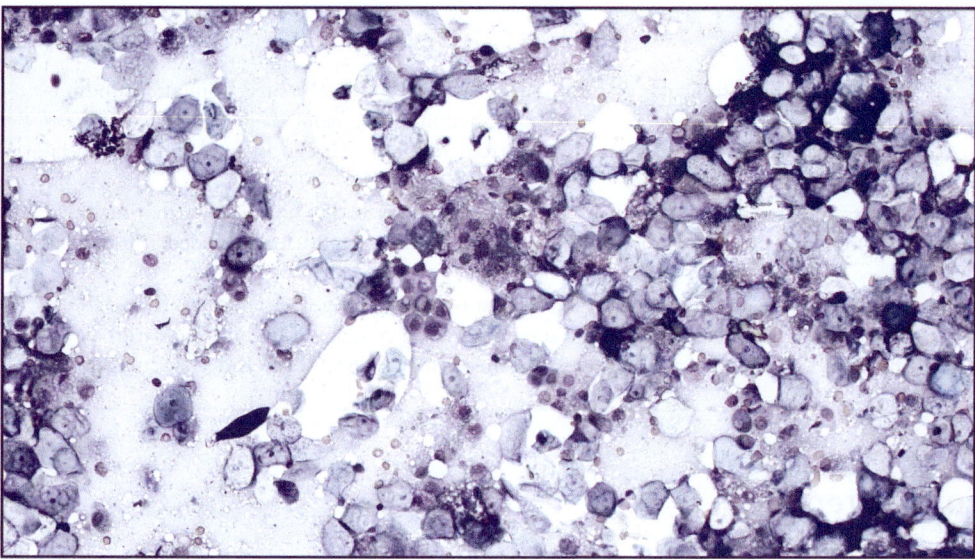

**Fig. 7.2.** Dog. Inflamed follicular cyst. Anucleated squames, cholesterol crystals admixed with macrophages and a few neutrophils. Wright-Giemsa.

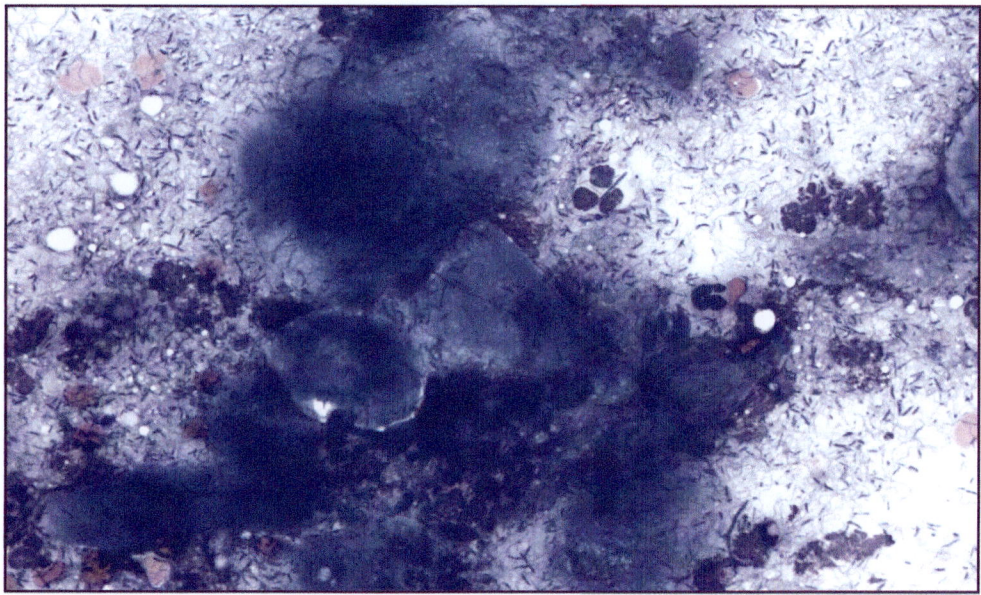

**Fig. 7.3.** Dog. Infected follicular cyst. Anucleated squames with degenerate neutrophils and intracytoplasic bacteria. Wright-Giemsa

**Pearls and Pitfalls**

- As cytologically a follicular cyst cannot be definitively differentiated from an infundibular keratinizing acanthoma and trichoepithelioma, a general diagnosis of '*keratinized lesion*' or '*follicular lesion*' is usually preferred, and follicular cyst is listed as a differential diagnosis.
- A disseminated form of follicular cysts has been described in a case series that included five dogs and one cat. Numbers of lesions were more than 20 and exceeded 150–200 in three of the cases.
- Dermoid cysts are congenital anomalies that occur in young dogs and cats. They arise on the midline. They contain lamellar keratin, yielding cytological findings similar to an infundibular cyst. Over-represented canine breeds include Rhodesian Ridgeback and Boxer.

## Further reading

Adedeji, A.O., Affolter, V.K. and Christopher, M.M. (2017) Cytological features of cutaneous follicular tumours and cysts in dogs. *Veterinary Clinical Pathology* 43(2), 143–150.

White, A., Stern, A., Campbell, K. and Santoro, D. (2013) Multiple (disseminated) follicular cysts in five dogs and one cat. *Veterinary Record* 173(11), 269.

## 7.2 (Sweat Gland) Apocrine Cyst

Non-neoplastic lesion lined by a single layer of apocrine secretory epithelial cells.

### Clinical features
- Relatively common in dogs; rare in cats.
- Age: 6 years or older.
- In dogs, it predominantly occurs on the head, legs, neck and trunk. In cats, it is often observed on the head.
- Cysts are usually solitary, occasionally multiple (apocrine cystomatosis). They are variably sized, well defined and fluctuant. They may have a blue tint when viewed through the overlying skin. Cyst content is usually clear and watery, but is occasionally brown and gelatinous due to inspissation.
- It is a benign lesion and carries a good prognosis.
- Over-represented breeds:
  - Dogs: Old English Sheepdog and Weimaraner.
  - Cats: Persian cat.

### Cytological features
- Background: generally clear. It may contain cholesterol crystals.
- Aspirates may be acellular or contain low numbers of macrophages.
- Cuboidal apocrine epithelial cells rarely exfoliate (for morphology, refer to 'Sweat gland adenoma and carcinoma' in section 8.5, Apocrine Gland Tumours).
- Following trauma, a variable degree of haemorrhage can occur within the cyst. In this case, macrophages may display erythrophagia or contain haemosiderin granules and/or haematoidin crystals.

---

**Differential diagnosis**

Cystic apocrine adenoma

---

**Pearls and Pitfalls**

Variants of apocrine cyst are the ceruminous gland cysts in the inner pinnae and ear canal. These are more common in adult cats, especially in Abyssinian and Persian cats. These lesions appear as multiple, often numerous, nodules or vesicles. They are often dark in colour and may be mistaken clinically for melanocytic or vascular neoplasms.

## 7.3   Fibroadnexal Hamartoma

Developmental anomaly of the pilosebaceous unit. It may contain apocrine glands.

### Clinical features
- Reported in dogs and accounting for 1.7–2.7% of all cutaneous lesions.
- It is observed in middle-aged or older dogs.
- It may be secondary to chronic trauma and/or scar tissue formation, both resulting in entrapment and subsequent distortion of the adnexal structures. A primary defect of the pilosebaceous units cannot be excluded.
- Hamartomatous lesions can originate from follicles, collagen or from sebaceous glands. However, the coexistence of more adnexal structures is usually observed, hence the term fibroadnexal hamartoma.
- Solitary, firm, circumscribed and nodular to polypoid, dermal mass of variable sizes. It may extend to the subcutaneous tissue. The lesion may also be pigmented, alopecic and ulcerated.
- Fibroadnexal hamartoma is observed more frequently on the distal legs, especially on pressure points. Head and trunk may also be affected.
- It is a benign lesion and carries a good prognosis.
- Over-represented canine breeds: large breed dogs, in particularly Labrador Retriever but also Basset Hound, Maremma Sheepdog and Bracco Italiano.

### Cytological features
- Cellularity: generally very low.
- Background: clear to lightly basophilic, with variable degree of haemodilution. Keratin bars are frequently seen.
- Several of the following components may simultaneously be observed:
  - Small clusters of mature sebocytes (for morphology, refer to 'Sebaceous adenoma' in section 8.4, Sebaceous Tumours).
  - Small clusters of sweat gland apocrine epithelial cells (for morphology, refer to 'Sweat gland adenoma and carcinoma' in section 8.5, Apocrine Gland Tumours).
  - Variable numbers of spindle-shaped stromal cells.
- Mixed inflammation may be present.

---

**Differential diagnoses**
- Sebaceous adenoma/hyperplasia (when the sebaceous component prevails)
- Follicular hamartoma
- Trichofolliculoma

**Pearls and Pitfalls**

- Due to their nature, these lesions tend to be poorly exfoliative and cytology is often unrewarding. A definitive diagnosis is usually made on histopathology.
- Follicular hamartoma is rare and occurs more frequently in younger dogs. It is composed of aggregates of enlarged primary follicles, hyperplastic sebaceous glands and may be associated with a variable amount of stroma.
- Trichofolliculoma is a rare benign follicular neoplasm. It may exfoliate cuboidal epithelial cells (basaloid follicular epithelial cells), sebocytes, anucleated squamous epithelial cells and slender stromal cells. Hair shafts may also be seen.

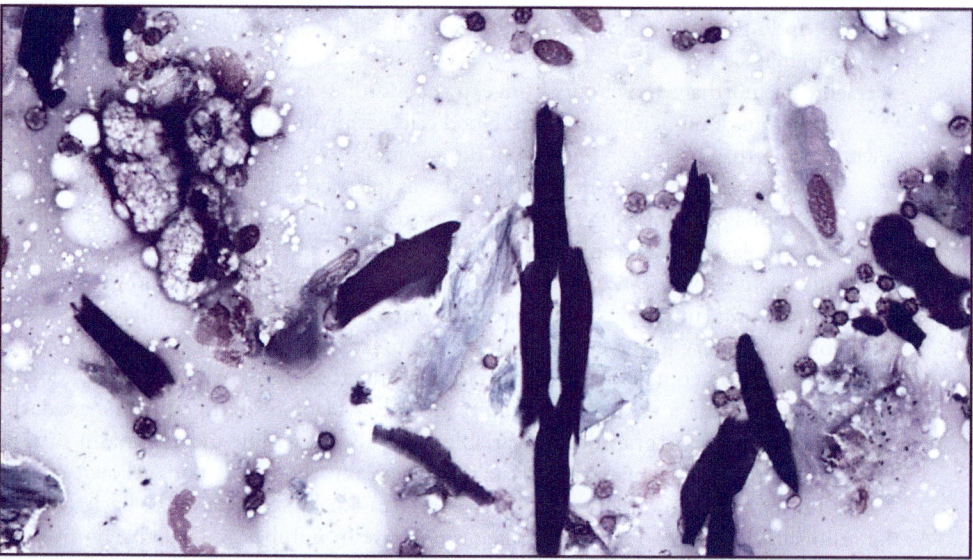

**Fig. 7.4.** Dog. Fibroadnexal hamartoma. Keratin bars, a few clusters of mature sebocytes and rare stromal mesenchymal cells. Wright-Giemsa.

## 7.4  Haematoma and Haemorrhage

A haematoma is an abnormal collection of blood outside a blood vessel secondary to haemor-rhage. Haemorrhage is an escape of blood from a ruptured blood vessel.

### Clinical features
- Organizing haematoma appears as a discrete cutaneous and subcutaneous mass. It can be cavitated and often contains variable amounts of blood.

### Cytological features
- Cytological findings depend on the time of onset of the haematoma/haemorrhage at the time of sampling:
  - Peracute haemorrhage (few hours from extravasation):
    - Background: numerous intact red blood cells with/without platelets.
  - Acute haemorrhage (> 12–24 hours from extravasation):
    - Background: numerous intact red blood cells (platelets will be dissolved by this time)
    - Macrophages displaying erythrophagocytosis: intact red blood cells are seen within the cytoplasm of macrophages.
  - Chronic haemorrhage (> 24–36 hours from extravasation):
    - Background: numerous red blood cells, intact or lysed. Cholesterol crystals may form secondary to the erythrocyte membrane dissolution.
    - Macrophages containing the degradation products of the red blood cell breakdown (haemosiderin and/or haematoidin crystals). Haemosiderin appears as dark basophilic-black granules of variable sizes, always within the cytoplasm of the macrophages. Haematoidin crystals are typically rhomboid and yellow/orange. They may be found in the macrophages or occasionally scattered in the background.
- As the lesion starts to organize, macrophages increase in number and reactive fibroblasts are often seen. Other inflammatory cell types may also be present.

### Causes
- Trauma.
- Vascular neoplasms (haemangioma and haemangiosarcoma) or any other poorly exfoliative neoplasms associated with local haemorrhage.

**Differential diagnosis**
Vascular neoplasms

**Pearls and Pitfalls**

- Cytological differentiation between haematoma and poorly exfoliative vascular neoplasms is often not possible based on cytology alone. Final diagnosis requires histopathology.
- In cases of aspiration of fluid, erythrophagocytosis may occur *in vitro*, as a result of delayed sample preparation.
- Haemosiderin can slightly vary in colour and, on certain occasions, may be difficult to distinguish from other granules, including melanin. Haemosiderin can be confirmed by using Prussian blue.
- Haematoidin is a haemoglobin product biochemically similar to bilirubin, which can be extracellular and/or intracellular. It forms when haemorrhage occurs in a closed tissue compartment and is the result of haemoglobin metabolism under low oxygen tension conditions. Following erythrocyte degeneration, haemoglobin is converted to porphyrin and then to biliverdin. The latter is reduced to crystalline haematoidin. As haematoidin can be converted back to biliverdin, it is not always seen.

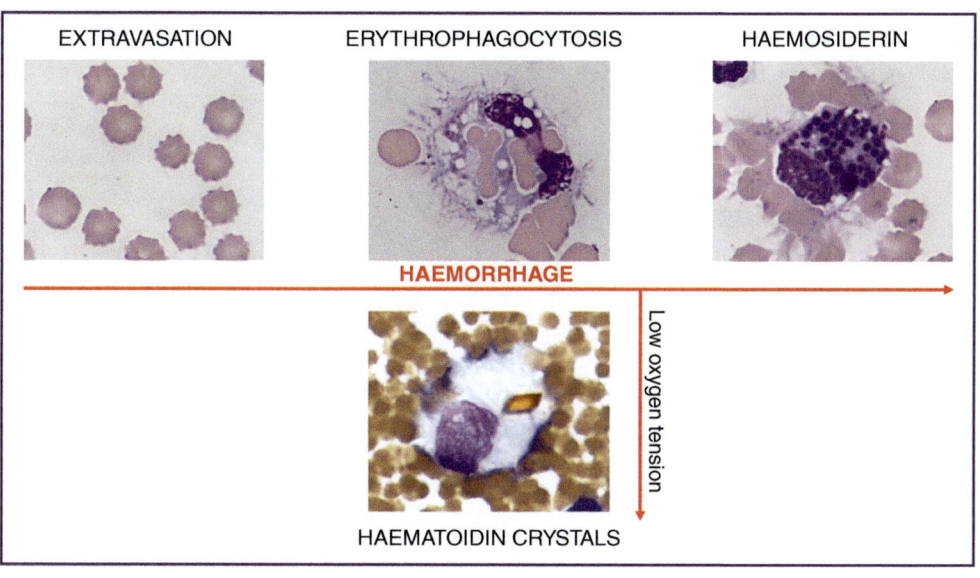

**Fig. 7.5.** Cytological changes expected in association with haemorrhage. Wright-Giemsa.

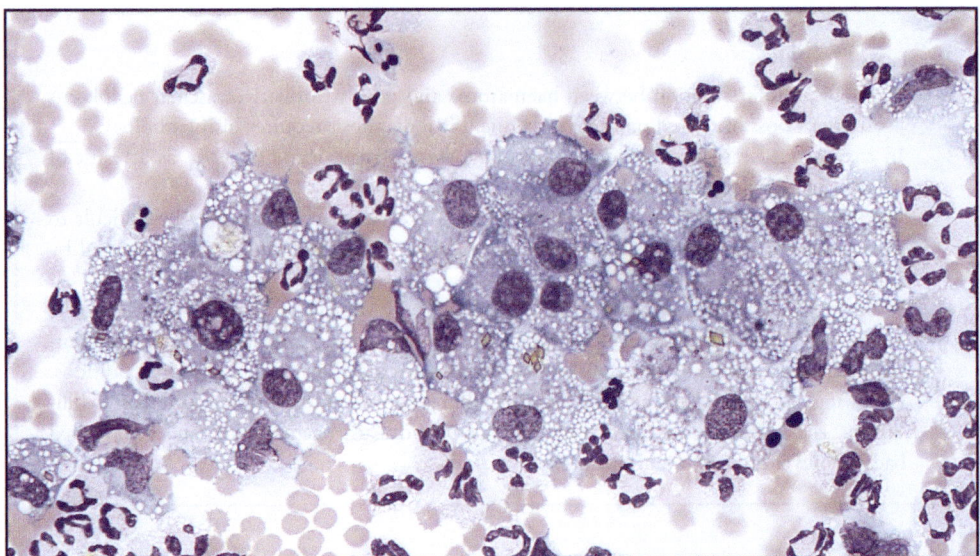

**Fig. 7.6.** Dog. Haemorrhage. Vacuolated macrophages containing rhomboid haematoidin crystals. Wright-Giemsa.

## 7.5 Necrosis

End-stage tissue injury that results in cell death.

### Clinical features

- Necrosis in skin and subcutis is more frequently seen in association with:
    - Fast-growing tumours.
    - Haematoma/haemorrhage.
    - Trauma to the adipose tissue.
- Necrosis is characterized by the loss of cytoplasmic and nuclear membrane integrity leading to influx of water into the cells, denaturation of intracellular proteins and digestion of the injured cells.
- Necrosis typically evokes a strong inflammatory response.

## Cytological findings

- Cellularity: variable.
- Background: generally contains a large amount of basophilic amorphous material, which represents the cytoplasmic and nuclear debris of the dead cells. Cholesterol crystals may be present.
- When associated with neoplasia, variable numbers of neoplastic cells can be found amongst the necrotic material. They may have a variable degree of degeneration and cellular details are usually lost.
- There is often a background of lysed erythrocytes with products of red blood cell degradation, such as haemosiderin and haematoidin.
- Necrotic adipose tissue, when present, is characterized by collapsed adipocytes, which tend to have more basophilic (blue-green) colour compared with viable adipocytes.
- Neutrophils and macrophages are frequently present in association with necrosis. Neutrophils are often degenerate, displaying nuclear and cytoplasmic swelling (karyolysis), also in absence of infection. Macrophages often contain amorphous phagosomes.

## Causes

- Hypoxaemia and ischaemia due to inappropriate tissue vascularization in fast-growing tumours.
- Irritants.
- Trauma.

### Pearls and Pitfalls

The centre of large and fast-growing masses is often necrotic. Hence, sampling from more peripheral areas should increase the probability of obtaining a representative and diagnostic sample.

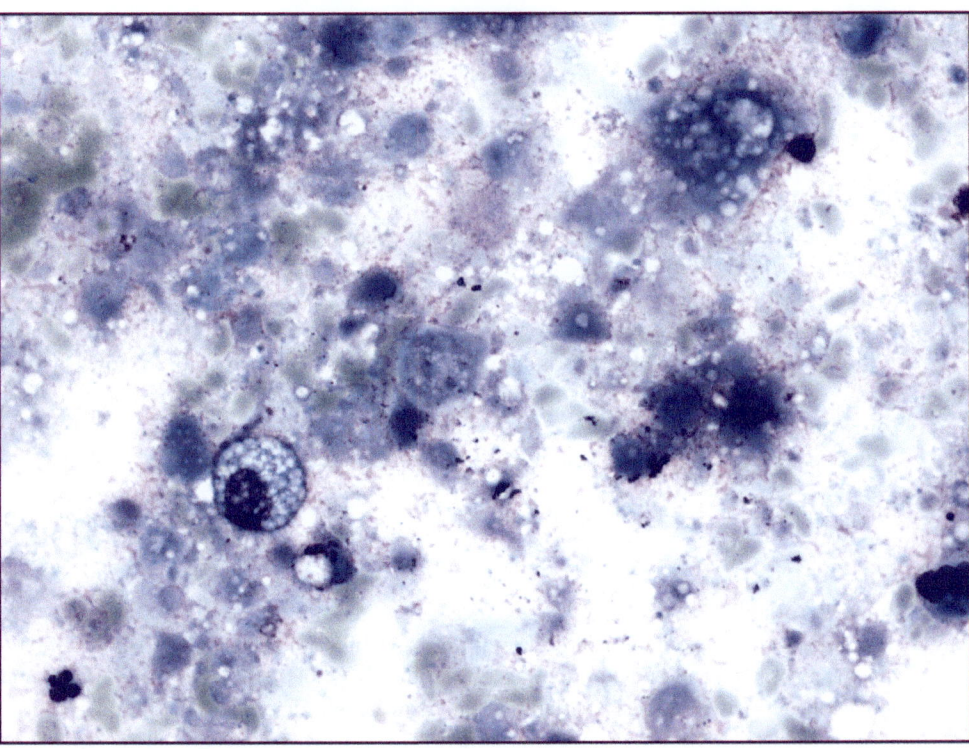

**Fig. 7.7.** Dog. Necrosis secondary to fast-growing neoplasia. The background contains a large amount of basophilic amorphous material. One vacuolated macrophage is present. Wright-Giemsa.

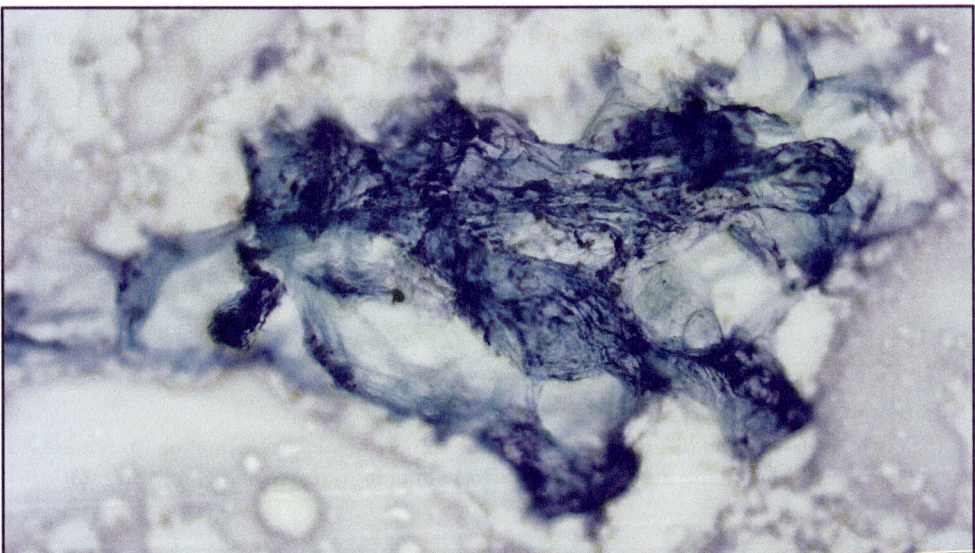

**Fig. 7.8.** Dog. Fat necrosis. Group of collapsed necrotic adipocytes. Note the blue-green colour of the cytoplasmic membrane. Wright-Giemsa.

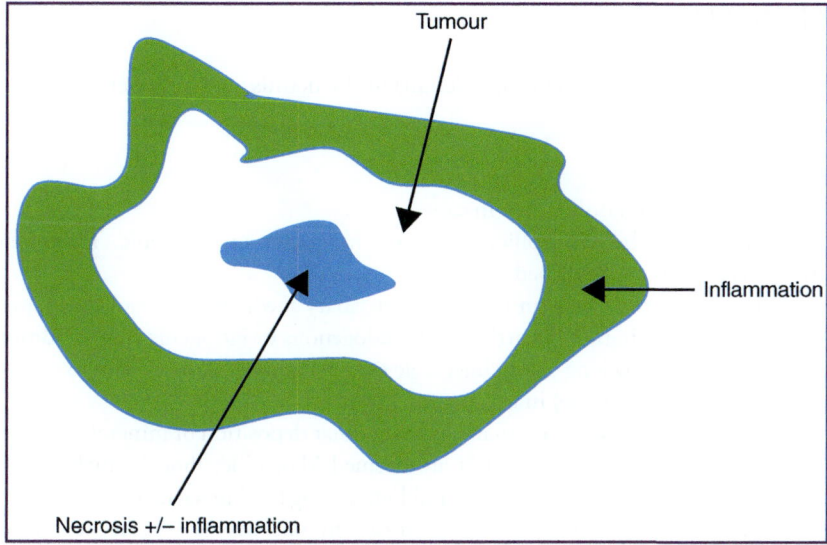

**Fig. 7.9.** The centre of fast-growing tumours is often necrotic and variably inflamed. Sampling from more peripheral areas should guarantee a more representative sample.

## 7.6 Calcinosis

Deposition of mineral (mostly containing calcium) in the dermis, and/or subcutis.

### Clinical features

- Reported in dogs and only rarely in cats.
- Mineralization can be dystrophic, metastatic, idiopathic or iatrogenic. Three major forms of calcinosis are described:
  - Calcinosis cutis: this term is used in veterinary medicine to denote widespread dermal mineralization occurring with endogenous or iatrogenic steroid administration (especially long-acting injectable corticosteroids). It may evolve to osteoma cutis (metaplastic bone) in late stages.
  - Calcinosis circumscripta: usually focal, nodular deposition of mineral salts in the subcutaneous tissue. Most cases are deemed idiopathic, though might be dystrophic secondary to focal trauma and long-lasting local ischaemia.
  - Systemic mineralization: deposition of calcium salts may also occur secondary to renal failure, underlying neoplasms or it may be iatrogenic secondary to injection of calcium-based products.
- Single or multiple pale yellow to white papules, plaques, or nodules, often coalescing and releasing gritty white material upon aspiration. These may become ulcerated and infected. Calcinosis circumscripta mostly presents as a single, well defined, subcutaneous nodule.
- Anatomical locations are variable:
  - Calcinosis cutis: observed more often in skin regions subject to repetitive flexure.
  - Calcinosis circumscripta: observed at sites of potential trauma (e.g. pressure points, bone prominences), tongue and ears and in the paw pads secondary to renal disease.
  - Systemic mineralization: calcium salts tend to deposit in organs rich with negatively charged elastic fibres, such as lungs, stomach, but may also involve the skin. Prognosis is good after surgical excision of calcinosis cutis.
- Over-represented canine breeds:
  - Calcinosis cutis: Bulldog, Labrador Retriever, Rottweiler, Boxer and Staffordshire Bull Terrier (often secondary to iatrogenic hyperadrenocorticism).
  - Calcinosis circumscripta: young, rapidly growing large-breed dogs, especially German Shepherd and brachycephalic dogs, such as Boston Terrier and Boxer, which are predisposed to dystrophic and idiopathic forms.

### Cytological features

- Cellularity is generally low.
- Background: pale grey-basophilic with numerous variably small and irregularly shaped refractile structures with angular borders. These are better appreciated with a lowered microscope condenser.

- Inflammatory response of variable degree. Inflammatory cells are mostly macrophages, with low numbers of giant multinucleated cells and occasionally neutrophils. Neutrophils are more frequent in ulcerated lesions. Small lymphocytes and plasma cells may also be seen.
- Amorphous purple material (likely necrotic tissue) can be observed.
- Fibroblasts may be present, especially in calcinosis circumscripta.

**Differential diagnoses**

- Tissue necrosis
- Granulomatous inflammation of other aetiology

**Pearls and Pitfalls**

- Cytochemical stains (von Kossa and Alizarin red S) can be used to confirm the presence of calcium deposits and may be required in hypercellular samples where the inflammatory component prevails and the crystals are hardly detectable on regular microscopy.
- The addition of immersion oil to the slide generally causes a characteristic change in the colour of the background.

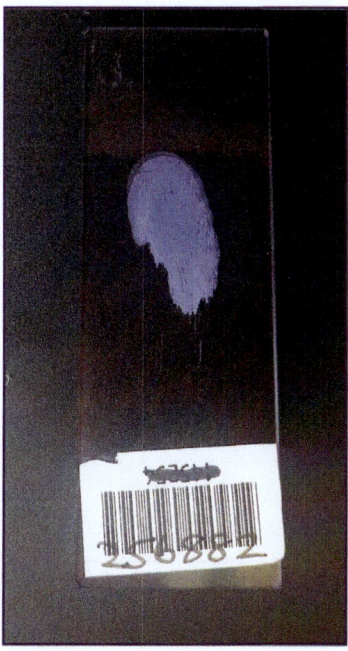

**Fig. 7.10.** Dog. Calcinosis. Appearance of a stained cytological smear of calcinosis. Note the characteristic chalky lavender colour.

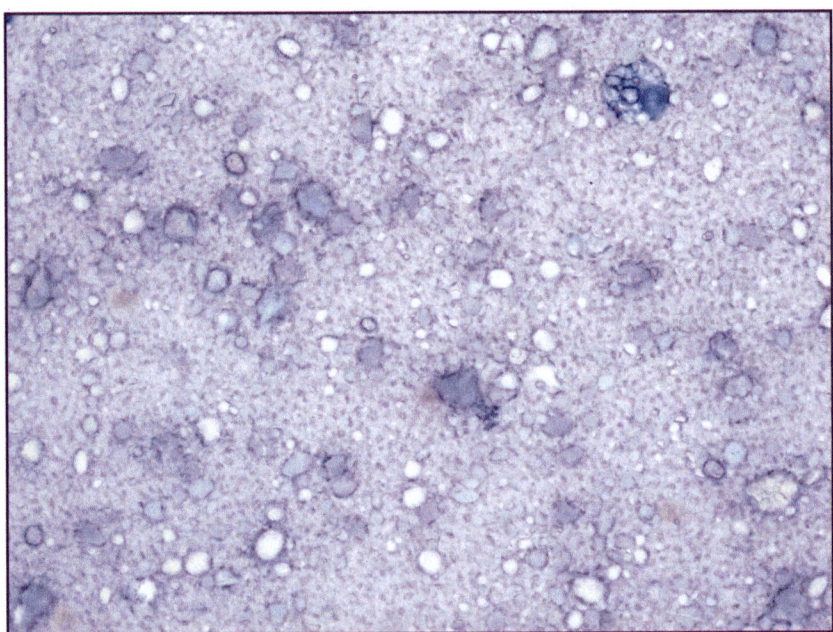

**Fig. 7.11.** Dog. Calcinosis. Mineral salts in the background admixed with rare macrophages. Wright Giemsa.

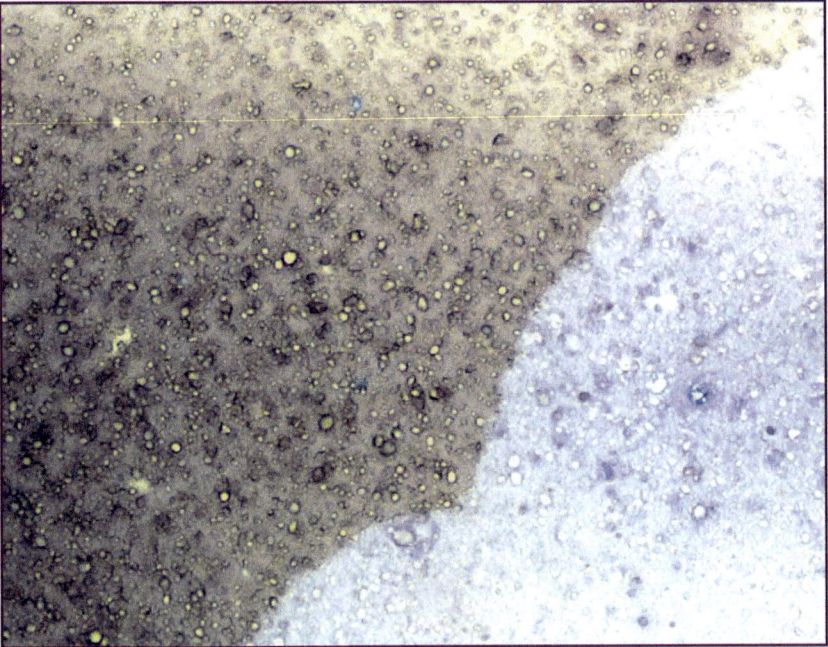

**Fig. 7.12.** Dog. Calcinosis. Addition of immersion oil to the slide causing a characteristic change in the colour of the background. Wright Giemsa.

## Further reading

Doerr, K.A., Outerbridge, C.A., White, S.D., Kass, P.H., Shiraki, R., Lam, A.T. and Affolter, V.K. (2013) Calcinosis cutis in dogs: histopathological and clinical analysis of 46 cases. *Veterinary Dermatology* 24(3), 355–379.

## 7.7 Granulation Tissue

New connective tissue and blood vessels that form during the wound healing process.

### Clinical features
- Variable clinical presentation, from thick plaque to distinct, solid nodules. It may be ulcerated, inflamed and/or alopecic.
- It may be present anywhere in the body, at sites of previous trauma or surgery.

## Cytological features
- Cellularity is often low, unless inflamed.
- Background: clear or pale basophilic with a variable degree of haemodilution.
- Variable numbers of spindle cells, either individual or forming loose aggregates with a storiform arrangement. They are occasionally seen associated with small capillaries.
- Nuclei are generally small to medium sized, oval, occasionally folded. They have granular chromatin and occasionally visible nucleoli.
- The cytoplasm is moderate in amount, moderately basophilic, elongated, occasionally vacuolated or rarely containing small pink-purple granules.
- Cytological features of atypia are variable.
- Inflammatory cells of various types may be present.

**Differential diagnosis**

Soft tissue sarcoma

**Pearls and Pitfalls**

Differentiation between granulation tissue and mesenchymal neoplasia is easier on histopathology than cytology. Regular granulation tissue shows a transition from large pleomorphic cells centrally to more mature fibrocytes peripherally. Moreover, in granulation tissue, fibroblasts and capillaries are lined up perpendicularly to each other.

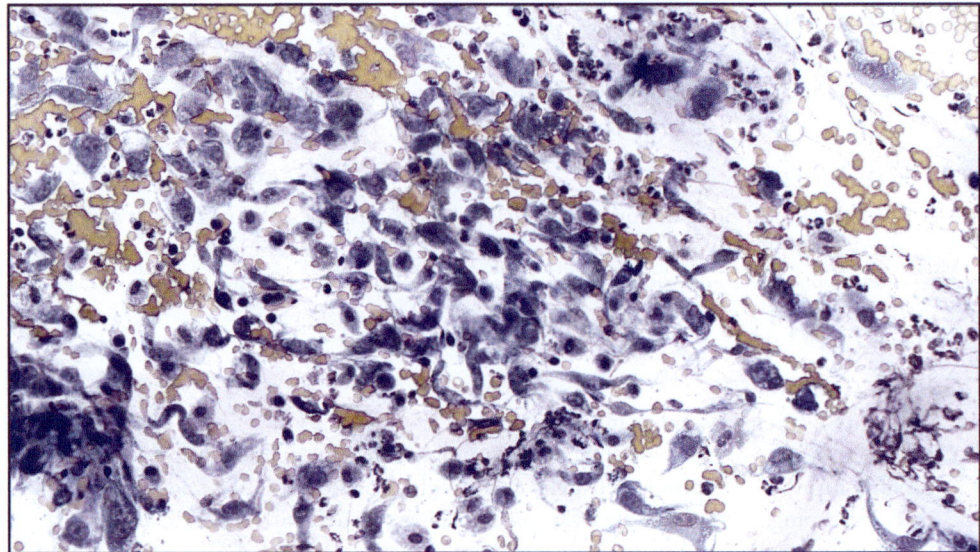

**Fig. 7.13.** Dog. Granulation tissue. Wright-Giemsa.

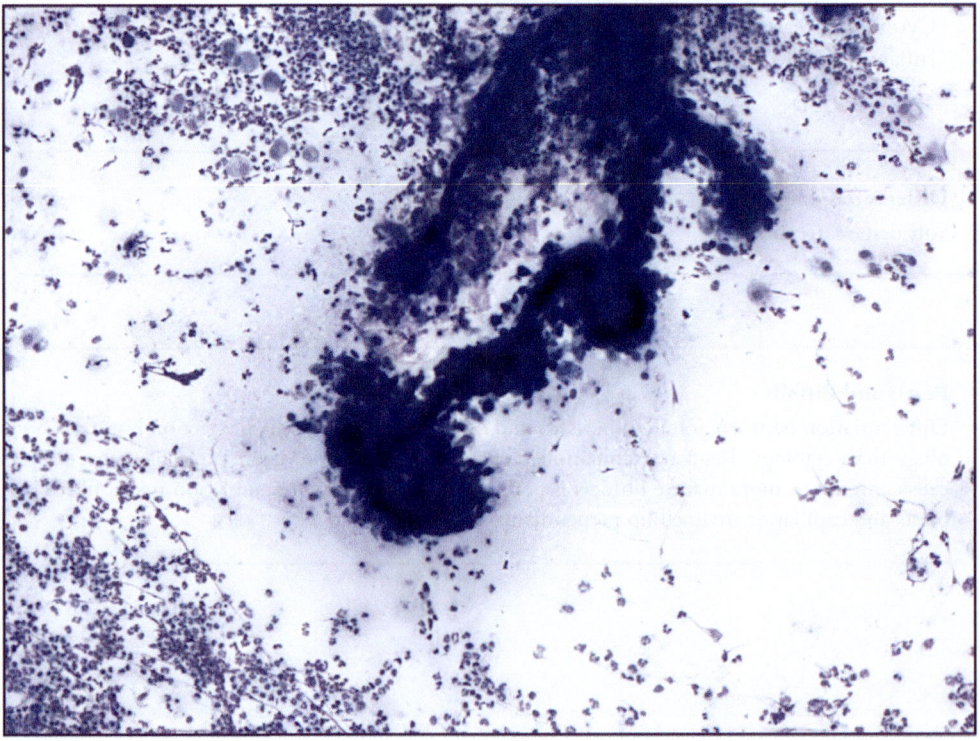

**Fig. 7.14.** Dog. Granulation tissue. Wright-Giemsa.

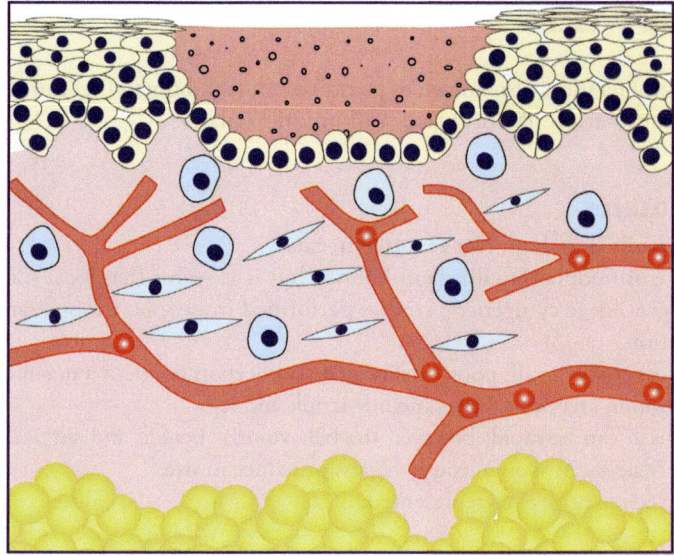

**Fig. 7.15.** Granulation tissue, graphical representation (Courtesy of Nic Ilchyshyn, DWR Diagnostics, UK).

# 7.8 Nodular Fasciitis

Non-neoplastic proliferation, also known as pseudosarcoma in human literature. Characterized by exuberant proliferation of fibroblasts and myofibroblasts.

## Clinical features
- Rarely described in dogs. Not reported in cats.
- The cause of nodular fasciitis is unknown, but it is seems that local trauma might be a trigger. Some cytogenetic studies performed in people demonstrated a clonal proliferation.
- Masses are variably sized, poorly delineated and deep in the derma or subcutis.
- Most common anatomical sites include trunk and legs.
- Mass growth can be rapid; however, the behaviour is benign and surgical excision is curative. Masses can spontaneously regress or reduce in size.
- Collie breeds may be over-represented.

## Cytological features
- Cellularity: generally high.
- Background: often characterized by the presence of a large amount of granular to fibrillar, pink amorphous material scattered throughout the slides and admixed with the cells. Haemo-dilution is variable and windrowing of the erythrocytes may be observed.
- Aspirates often contain numerous spindle cells arranged in medium-large aggregates or occasionally individualized.
- Nuclei are medium-large, round to oval. They have coarsely stippled to granular chromatin and may contain one to multiple, small to medium-sized, round and variably prominent nucleoli.
- The cytoplasm forms one or two tails that project away from the nucleus. It is pale to moderately basophilic and can contain small clear vacuoles or pink granules. Cell margins are generally poorly defined.
- Cellular pleomorphism is variable. Anisokaryosis and anisocytosis can be moderate. Occasional binucleation can be observed and rare mitoses found.
- In spite of the name that implies inflammation, inflammatory cells are not always observed. When present, they mostly consist of lymphocytes, plasma cells and histiocytes–macrophages.

**Differential diagnosis**

Sarcoma

**Pearls and Pitfalls**

Nodular fasciitis is an unusual benign lesion that mimics a malignant sarcomatous proliferation clinically, cytologically and, in some aspects, histopathologically. Cytology can only raise the suspicion of nodular fasciitis and histopathology is always required for the diagnosis. The cytological experience on this lesion is limited in the veterinary field and insufficient numbers of cases are available in literature to be able to identify specific features that may help in diagnosing nodular fasciitis. However, the presence of diffuse abundant granular eosinophilic background might be one of these (authors' observation), especially in the context of a young animal with history of trauma. Clinically and histopathologically, nodular fasciitis shares many similarities with nodular episcleritis.

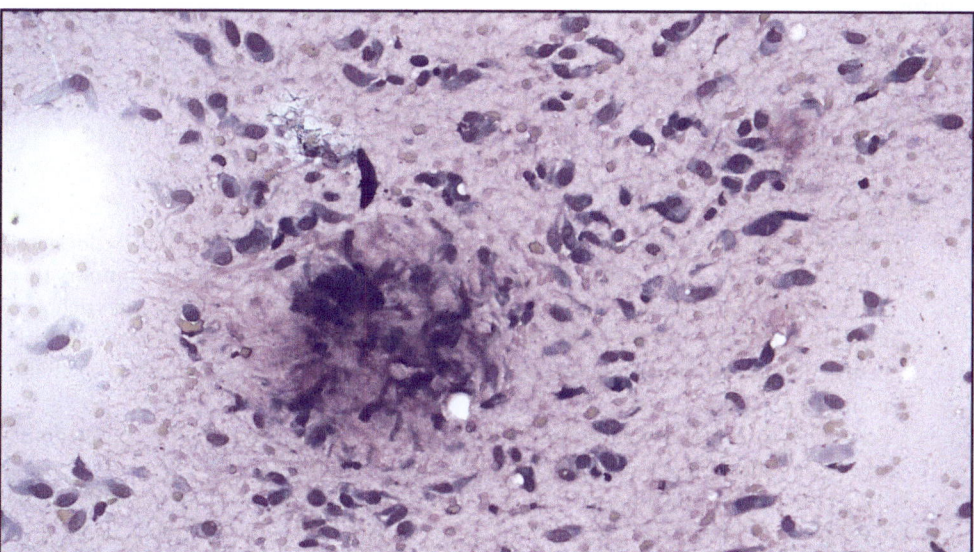

**Fig. 7.16.** Dog. Nodular fasciitis. Wright-Giemsa.

# 8 Epithelial Tumours

Cutaneous epithelial neoplasms can originate from any of the epithelial structures present in the skin and are classified based on the cell of origin and presence or absence of squamous or adnexal differentiation. The subcutaneous tissue lacks epithelial structures. Hence, there are no primary epithelial tumours arising in the subcutis. Cutaneous epithelial tumours can be broadly classified as follows:

- Epithelial tumours without squamous or adnexal differentiation:
    - Basal cell tumour.
- Tumours of the epidermis:
    - Papilloma.
    - Squamous cell carcinoma.
- Adnexal tumours:
    - Follicular tumours: different types of follicular tumours can be observed in dogs and cats, some of which cannot be differentiated on cytology. The follicular tumours that will be described in the specific sections of this book include: trichoblastoma, trichoepithelioma, pilomatricoma, and infundibular keratinizing acanthoma. These tumours, besides being the most frequent, may show some cytological features that facilitate their recognition on cytology.
    - Sebaceous and modified sebaceous glands tumours: sebaceous adenoma, epithelioma and carcinoma, and perianal gland adenoma, epithelioma and carcinoma.
    - Apocrine and modified apocrine glands tumours: sweat gland adenoma and carcinoma, anal sac adenocarcinoma, and ceruminous adenoma and carcinoma.
    - Adnexal tumours without further differentiation: clear cell adnexal carcinoma.

Merkel cell tumour will also be described in this section, although this is not strictly an epithelial tumour but a neuroendocrine neoplasm originating from mechanoreceptors present in the epidermis and follicular epithelium.

## Cytological diagnosis of cutaneous epithelial lesions

A practical approach to the cytological diagnosis of skin lesions (tumours or non-neoplastic epithelial lesions) should try to answer to the following questions:

- From what type of structure does the lesion originate (e.g. epidermis, sebaceous or sweat glands, hair follicle)?
- Is the lesion benign or malignant?
- Less frequently, is it a primary cutaneous neoplasm or a cutaneous metastasis of another malignancy?

# Key cytological features

Some cutaneous epithelial tumours can exhibit an overlap of cellular and morphological features. In these cases, only a sub-classification is possible, leaving a list of main differential diagnoses. Some of the cytological findings that, when present, may help in distinguishing these cutaneous epithelial tumours from each other are as follows:

**Table 8.1**

Trichoblastoma (TB) versus basal cell tumour (BC)
- Ribbon-like arrangement (TB)
- Presence of pink amorphous material associated with the epithelial cells (TB)
- Stromal cells (TB)

Trichoblastoma (TB) versus trichoepithelioma (TE) and infundibular keratinizing acanthoma (IKA)
- Ribbon-like arrangement (TB)
- Presence of anucleated squamous epithelial cells (TE: large polygonal squames and/or ghost cells; IKA: large polygonal squames)
- Neutrophilic, pyogranulomatous or granulomatous inflammation (TE and IKA)

Trichoblastoma (TB) versus sweat gland adenoma (SA)
- Ribbon-like arrangement (TB)
- Presence of pink amorphous material associated with the epithelial cells (TB)
- Tubular arrangement (rarely seen on cytology) (SA)
- Columnar epithelial cells (SA)
- Possible presence of anucleated squamous epithelial cells (SA)
- Cytoplasmic granules of secretory material (SA)

Trichoepithelioma (TE) versus infundibular keratinizing acanthoma (IKA)
- Progressive maturation of the cells from cuboidal to superficial anucleated squamous epithelial cells (IKA)
- Ghost cells (TE)

Trichoepithelioma (TE) and infundibular keratinizing acanthoma (IKA) versus pilomatricoma (PM)
- Predominance of ghost cells (PM)
- Large polytonal anucleated squamous epithelial cells (TE and IKA)

In other epithelial neoplasms, specific cytological features are present, allowing the identification of the structure of origin and a more detailed diagnosis. For example, amongst the adnexal epithelial tumours, sebaceous and perianal gland neoplasms are those with the more characteristic morphological features that enable the cytologist to reach a definitive diagnosis of the lineage of the tumour.

# 8.1 Tumours without Squamous or Adnexal Differentiation

## Basal cell tumour and basal cell carcinoma

Tumours that originate from the basal cells of the epidermis and do not show squamous or adnexal differentiation.

### Clinical features

Following the 1998 World Health Organization (WHO) classification system, all tumours that were previously diagnosed as basal cell tumours were reclassified as either trichoblastomas or sweat gland adenomas. The new classification published by the David-Thompson DVM Foundation (Goldschmidt *et al.*, 2018) has reintroduced this tumour as a separate entity. Due to this, little is known about the true incidence, presentation and clinical behaviour of this tumour nowadays. The clinical information described below goes back to the studies performed before the 1998 WHO classification.

- Basal cell tumour (cats):
  - Benign tumour that arises from the basal cells of the epidermis.
  - Age: peak incidence between 6 and 13 years old.
  - Lesions are well circumscribed, can be alopecic, ulcerated and pigmented.
  - Most commonly reported on the head and neck.
  - Incomplete excision may result in tumour recurrence.
  - It is unknown if this tumour can progress to basal cell carcinoma.
- Basal cell carcinoma:
  - Age: peak incidence between 12 and 16 years old.
  - Usually appears as a thick plaque. It can be ulcerated and can infiltrate the dermis. It can be pigmented or non-pigmented.
  - Low-grade malignancy, thought to be rare in dogs and cats. Surgical excision is generally curative and metastases are very rare but have been reported.
  - Infiltrative forms may recur after surgical excision.
  - Over-represented feline breed: Ragdoll cat.

### Cytological features

- Cellularity is variable, generally moderate.
- Background: variably haemodiluted.
- The aspirates are composed of cuboidal epithelial cells in uniform and cohesive clusters, both seen in benign and malignant forms.
- Nuclei are small to medium sized and round. The chromatin is clumped and nucleoli are not seen.
- The cytoplasm is scant and moderately basophilic, often with indistinct borders. It often contains dark granules (melanin pigment).
- Anisokaryosis and anisocytosis are minimal in benign forms and could become more prominent in carcinomas. The N:C ratio is high.

**Differential diagnoses**

- Sweat gland adenoma
- Trichoblastoma
- Melanocytic tumour (when containing melanin)

**Pearls and Pitfalls**

- Basal cell tumours usually lack a significant stroma. The presence of slender spindle cells, especially if numerous, is more typical of trichoblastoma.
- Basal cell tumours are often pigmented and may be confused clinically and microscopically with melanocytic neoplasms.
- In dogs, tumours previously classified as basal cell tumours have now been reclassified as trichoblastomas.
- In cats, tumours previously classified as basal cell tumours that show a focal or multifocal ductal differentiation have been reclassified as aprocrine ductal adenomas.

## 8.2 Epidermal Tumours

### Papilloma

Benign proliferation of the epidermis that can be viral or non-viral in origin.

#### Clinical features
- Non-viral papilloma (squamous papilloma):
  - Age: no known age predisposition, though it is more frequently seen in old dogs.
  - Lesions are small, generally 1–5 mm and generally exophytic.
  - Most frequently localized on the face, eyelids, feet and conjunctiva.
  - It might be triggered by trauma.
  - Spontaneous regression is not expected.
- Viral papilloma (wart) (can be exophytic or inverted):
  - Exophytic papilloma: uncommon in dogs and rare in cats; single or multiple; frequent on face, ears and extremities.
  - Inverted papilloma: rare in dogs, usually younger than 3 years old; multiple and usually on ventral abdomen.
  - It can spontaneously regress within 6 weeks to 9 months.

#### Cytological features
- Cellularity is variable, often adequate.
- Background: variably haemodiluted.
- The aspirates are composed of large squamous epithelial cells that generally exfoliate individually.
- Cells are polygonal and angular with a low N:C ratio.
- Nuclei are round, central to paracentral. They are often large to very large and hyperchromatic. The chromatin is clumped and nucleoli are not seen.
- The cytoplasm is abundant and pale basophilic. Viral papillomas can contain bright fuchsia granulations and/or multiple small clear vacuoles. On histopathology, these cells are known as koilocytes and are typical but not pathognomonic of viral papillomas.
- Small lymphocytes and reactive fibroblasts may be seen in the regression phase.

**Differential diagnosis**
Squamous cell carcinoma (well-differentiated form)

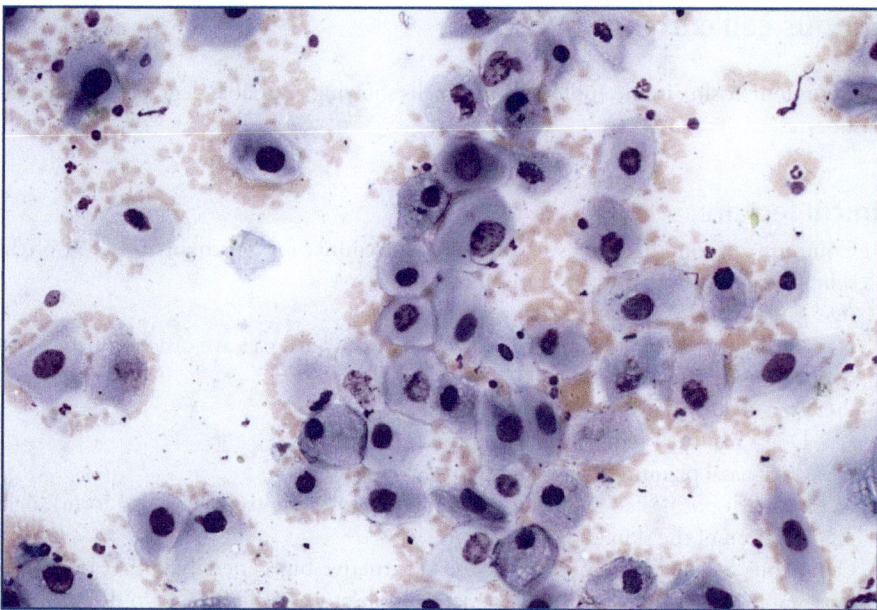

**Fig. 8.1.** Dog. Papilloma. There are numerous large squamous epithelial cells with large hyperchromatic nuclei and abundant dense and pale basophilic cytoplasm. Wright-Giemsa.

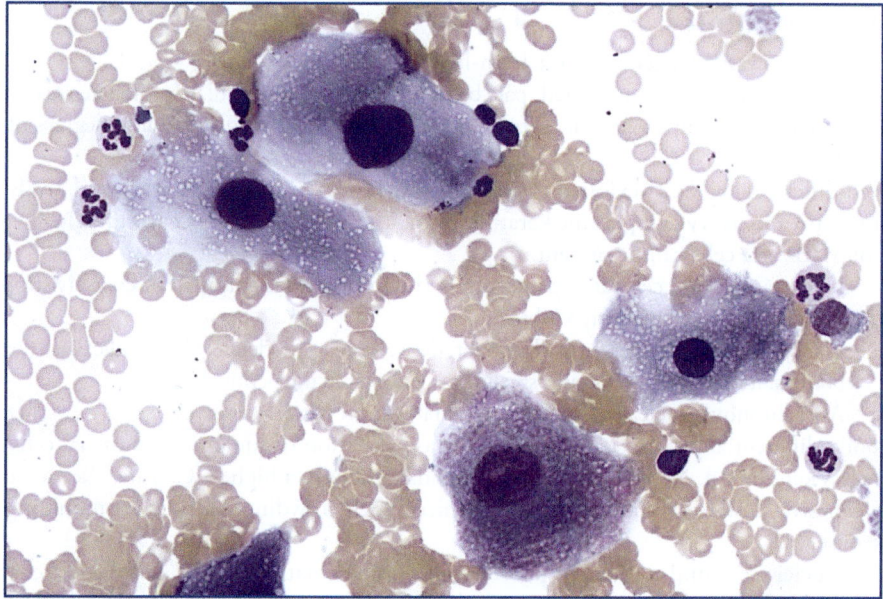

**Fig. 8.2.** Dog. Papilloma. Koilocyte-like cells in a viral papilloma. Some of the squamous epithelial cells have a vacuolar cytoplasm, others contain fuchsia granules. Wright-Giemsa.

## Further reading

Moore, A.R., Libby, A.L., Khanal, S., Ehrhart, E.J. and Avery, P. (2016) Is this cell hollow? *Veterinary Clinical Pathology* 45(1), 8–9.

Sprague, W. and Thrall, M.A. (2001) Recurrent skin mass from the digit of a dog. *Veterinary Clinical Pathology* 30(4), 189–192.

# Squamous cell carcinoma (SCC)

Malignant tumour arising in the epidermis, with cells showing a variable degree of differentiation to keratinocytes.

## Clinical features

- Common tumour in domestic animals. It accounts for approximately 5% of the skin tumours in dogs and 15% in cats.
- Age: 6–13 years in dogs and 9–14 years in cats.
- Usually solitary lesion, but multiple SCCs can occur. Masses are often alopecic, erythematous and ulcerated.
- Preferred anatomical sites:
  - Dogs: nail bed, scrotum, lips, ventral trunk and legs.
  - Cats: nasal planum, eyelids and pinnae.
- In cats, predisposing factors include chronic sun exposure (solar-induced form), light pigmentation of the skin and lack of hair.
- Cutaneous SCC is locally invasive and destructive but generally with a low metastatic rate. The highest metastatic tendency is observed in digit SCC in dogs.
- Metastases usually occur to the draining lymph node and rarely to other organs.

## Cytological features

- Cellularity is variable, generally medium-high.
- Background: variably haemodiluted, pale basophilic and finely granular (proteinaceous).
- The aspirates are composed of numerous squamous epithelial cells at variable degrees of differentiation.
- Well-differentiated SCC exfoliates polygonal squamous epithelial cells with a relatively low N:C ratio and heavy cytoplasmic keratinization. These cells usually occur individually or in groups. Bizarre cells can be present.
  - Nuclei are round, central to paracentral. The chromatin is clumped or coarsely stippled. Nucleoli are usually poorly visible.
  - The cytoplasm is moderate to abundant, dense, pale to moderately basophilic, with angular borders. It occasionally contains small, clear vacuoles in the perinuclear area.
  - Asynchronous nuclear to cytoplasmic maturation can be observed.
- Poorly differentiated SCC usually exfoliates a population of squamous epithelial cells that are less keratinized. Neoplastic cells are cuboidal and have a high N:C ratio. They are often in cohesive clusters, which may be disorganized. Cell crowding and nuclear moulding can be observed.
  - Nuclei are round, central to paracentral. The chromatin is finely clumped to coarsely stippled and multiple prominent nucleoli are often seen.
  - The cytoplasm is scant to moderate, moderately basophilic.
  - Mitoses may be found.
  - Irregularly shaped cells may be observed (e.g. tadpole cells).
- A prominent neutrophilic inflammation is often present, as a result of the ulceration that frequently accompanies these lesions.
- Neutrophils can be found within the cytoplasm of the neoplastic cells. This phenomenon is known as emperipolesis.

# Variants

Some of the variants listed below can be recognized on cytology (e.g. spindle cell variant) or their cytological presentation has been described in literature (acantholytic variant). The others require histopathology for recognition.

- Acantholytic squamous cell carcinoma:
  - Cytologically, this variant is characterized by a heterogeneous population of round to spindle-shaped cells that exfoliate individually or in small clusters.
  - Nuclei are round with finely stippled to hyperchromatic chromatin.
  - The cytoplasm is amphophilic and finely vacuolated.
- Spindle cell squamous cell carcinoma:
  - Rare variant of poorly differentiated SCC.
  - Cells vary from polygonal to spindle shaped.
  - Spindle-shaped cells have round to oval nuclei and two cytoplasmic tails that project away from each side of the nucleus.
  - The cytoplasm is dense, pale to moderately basophilic and often has well-defined margins.
  - A transition from the spindle-shaped cells and the more classical polygonal cells usually helps in the diagnosis.
- Verrucous and papillary variants:
  - Rare variants.
  - Cytologically they are not distinguishable from the more classical form of SCC.

---

**Differential diagnoses**
- Keratinizing basal cell carcinoma
- Basosquamous carcinoma
- Papilloma

---

**Pearls and Pitfalls**

In cats, a multicentric form of squamous cell carcinoma in situ has been described. The neoplastic cells are confined to the epidermis and do not invade through the basement membrane. This form is characterized by the presence of multifocal plaques or verrucous lesions that can occur at any site and with no relationship to sun exposure.

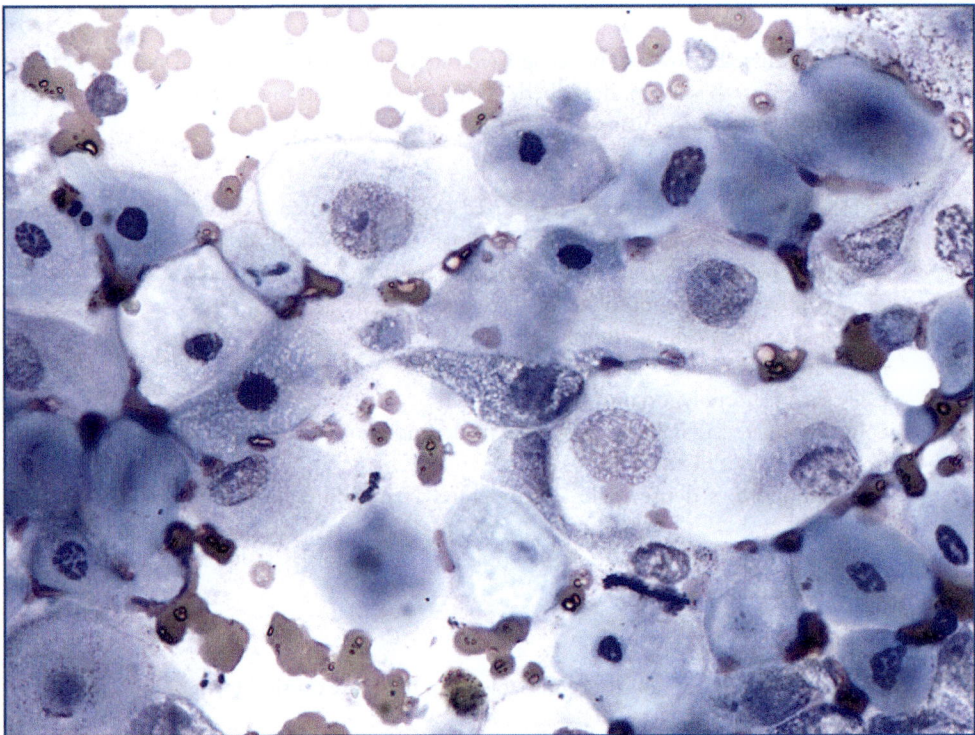

**Fig. 8.3.** Cat. Well-differentiated SCC. Wright-Giemsa.

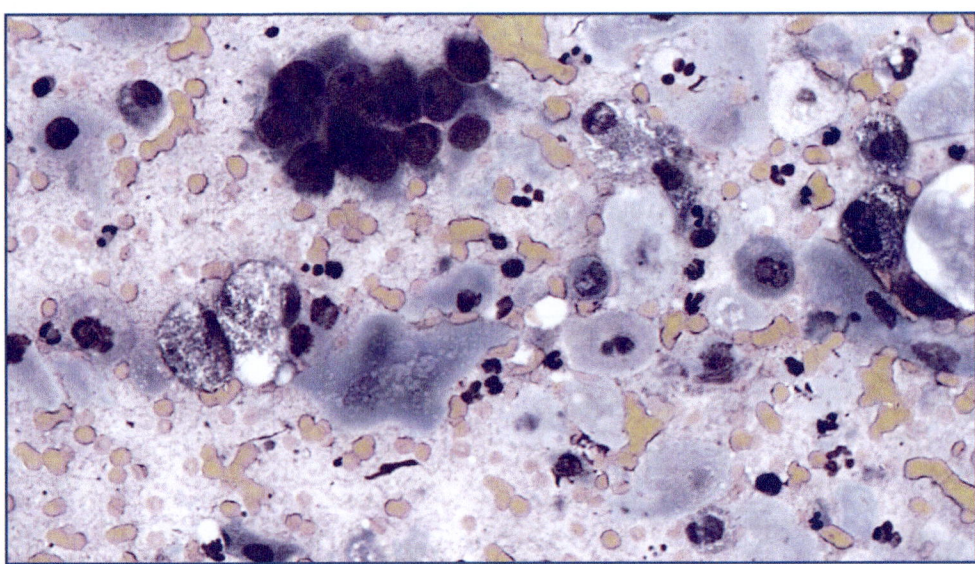

**Fig. 8.4.** Dog. Poorly differentiated SCC. Cuboidal nucleated cells with prominent nucleoli and high N:C ratio together with keratinized squamous epithelial cells. Wright-Giemsa.

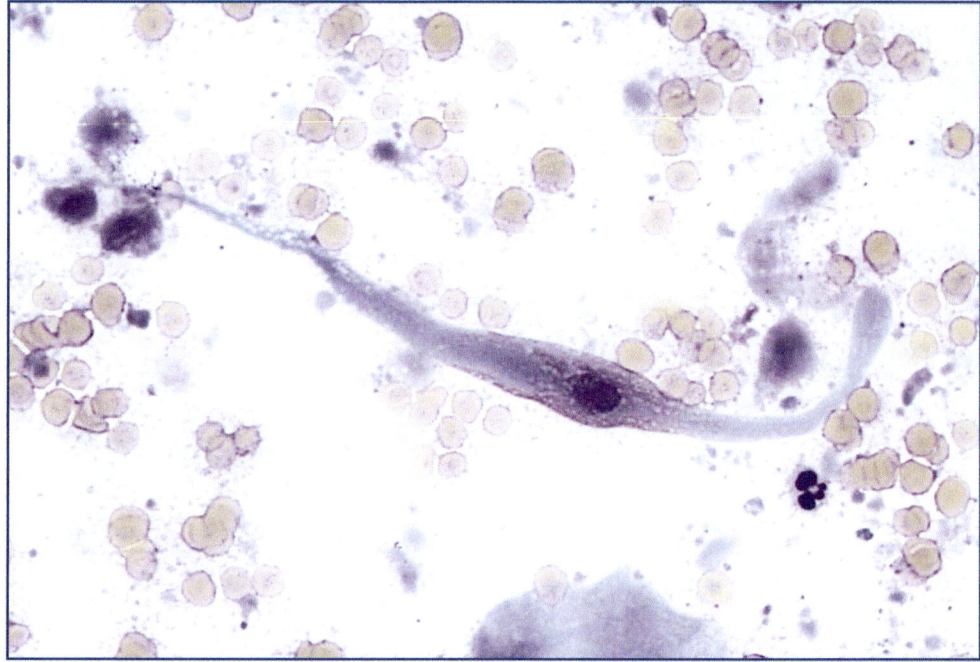

**Fig. 8.5.** Dog. SCC. Tadpole squamous epithelial cell. Wright-Giemsa.

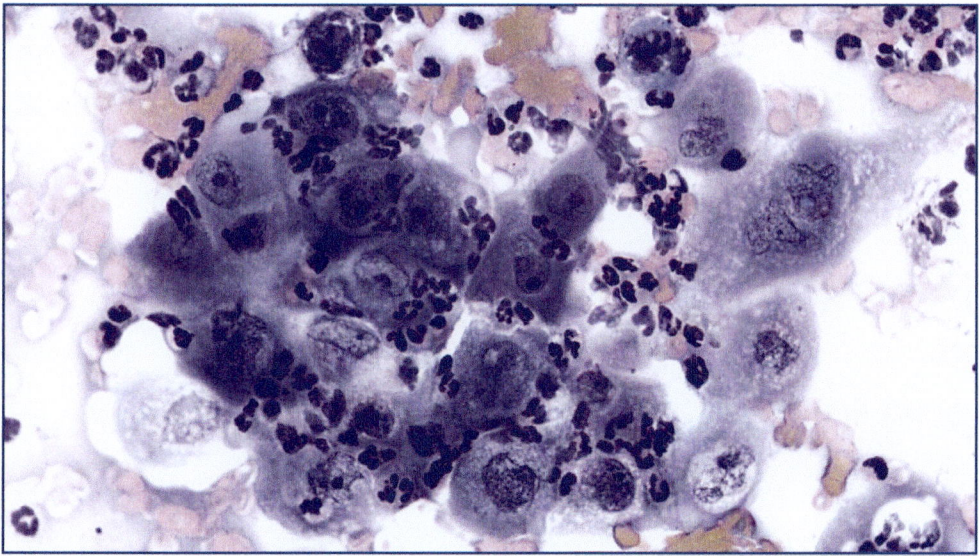

**Fig. 8.6.** Dog. SCC. Neoplastic squamous epithelial cells with intracytoplasmic neutrophils (emperipolesis). Wright Giemsa.

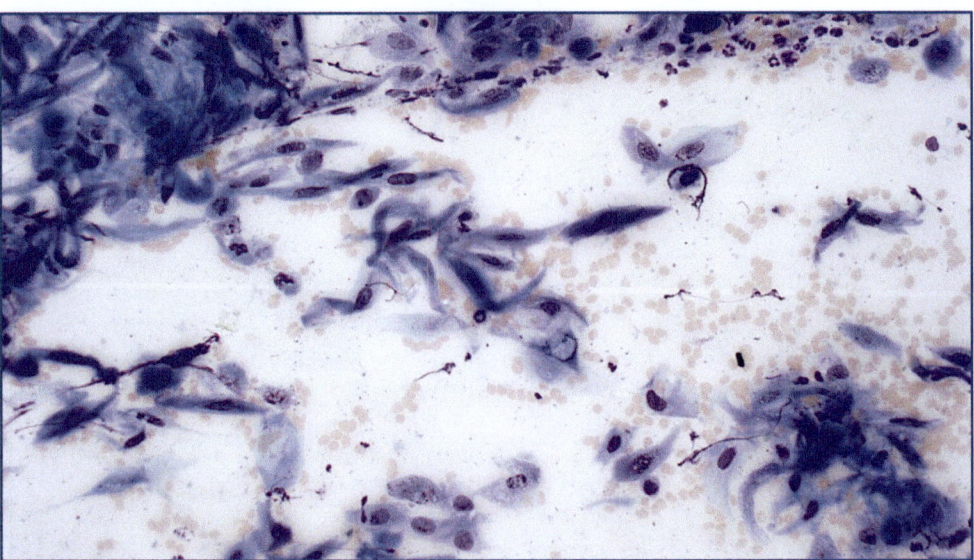

**Fig. 8.7.** Cat. Spindle cell variant of SCC. Wright-Giemsa.

## Further reading

Gradi, F., Monteriro, L.N., Fernandes, T.R., Salgado, B.S. and Rocha, N.S. (2011) What is your diagnosis? Cutaneous mass in the mammary region of a dog. *Veterinary Clinical Pathology* 40, 101–102.

# 8.3 Follicular Tumours

## Trichoblastoma

Benign tumour that derives or shows differentiation to the primitive hair germ cells.

### Clinical features
- Common tumour in dogs and fairly common in cats.
- Age in dogs: 4–10 years old.
- In dogs it generally presents as a solitary, firm and alopecic mass, polipoid or dome-shaped. In cats, masses are usually solitary and dome-shaped.
- In dogs, it more frequently occurs on the head, neck and at the base of the ears. In cats, it most frequently occurs on the head and cranial half of the trunk.
- Trichoblastoma carries a good prognosis; the malignant counterpart of trichoblastoma has never been described in dogs and cats, but it is rarely reported in people.

## Cytological features
- Cellularity is variable from low to high.
- Background: clear to lightly basophilic. Haemodilution is possible.
- Neoplastic cells are cuboidal and are arranged in variably sized cohesive and uniform clusters. Palisade arrangement is common.
- Nuclei are small to medium sized, with clumped chromatin and inconspicuous nucleoli.
- The cytoplasm is scant and lightly to moderately basophilic. It can contain a variable amount of melanin pigment.
- Anisokaryosis and anisocytosis are minimal.
- Cells can be associated with a small amount of extracellular pink amorphous material (possible basement membrane).
- Low to numeorus slender spindle cells can be found, often individually scattered in the background (stromal cells).

## Variants
- Ribbon and medusoid variants:
  - Both variants are common in dogs and rare in cats.
  - Cells are arranged in branching, winding and radiating columns (ribbons), generally two cells in width. The cell cords radiate from a central island in the medusoid type.
  - Cells are uniform and cuboidal. Cytoplasm is more abundant in the ribbon type.
- Granular cell variant:
  - Uncommon form in dogs and rare in cats.
  - Cells are individualized, medium to large and round to polygonal.
  - Nuclei are oval, eccentric, with smooth chromatin and an inconspicuous nucleolus.
  - The cytoplasm is abundant, has distinct borders and contains light purple granules.
  - Variable numbers of cuboidal epithelial cells may be present.

- Solid/cystic variant:
  - Reported rarely in dogs.
  - Masses are often multilobular. Lobules can have a central cyst delineated by small keratinocytes. Cysts contain pale basophilic proteinaceous material or black necrotic material.
  - Melanocytes may be present amongst the epithelial cells.
- Trabecular variant:
  - Multilobulated tumour, common in cats and rare in dogs.
  - Cells at the periphery of the tumour are in palisades and cuboidal. Cells in the centre of the neoplasm have slightly more cytoplasm.
  - Melanocytes can be found amongst the neoplastic cells, singly or in small groups.
- Spindle cell variant:
  - This variant is more common in cats and rare in dogs.
  - Cells are uniform, elongated and occur individually and in variably sized cohesive clusters.
  - Nuclei are small and cigar-shaped, with coarse chromatin and 1–2 small prominent nucleoli.
  - The cytoplasm is pale basophilic, elongated and with inconspicuous cell margins.

---

**Differential diagnoses**
- Basal cell tumour (cats)
- Sweat gland adenoma
- Sebaceous epithelioma (though sebocytes are usually seen)
- Melanocytoma (when trichoblastoma is heavily pigmented)
- Granular cell tumour (for the granular cell variant. However, granular cell tumour in skin is very rare in dogs and cats)

---

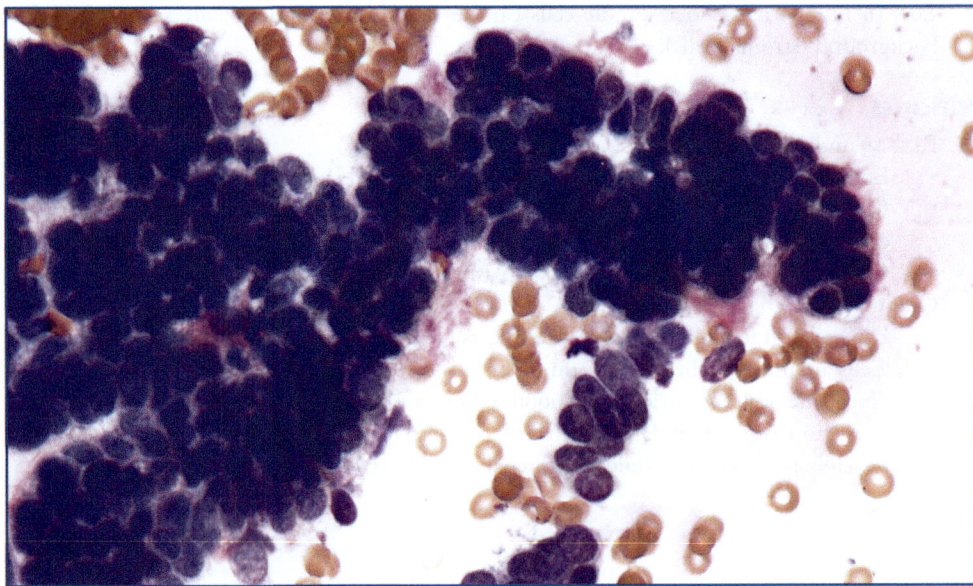

**Fig. 8.8.** Dog. Trichoblastoma. Uniform cuboidal epithelial cells. They show the typical arrangement in palisades. Cells are associated with a small amount of pink amorphous material (basement membrane). Wright-Giemsa.

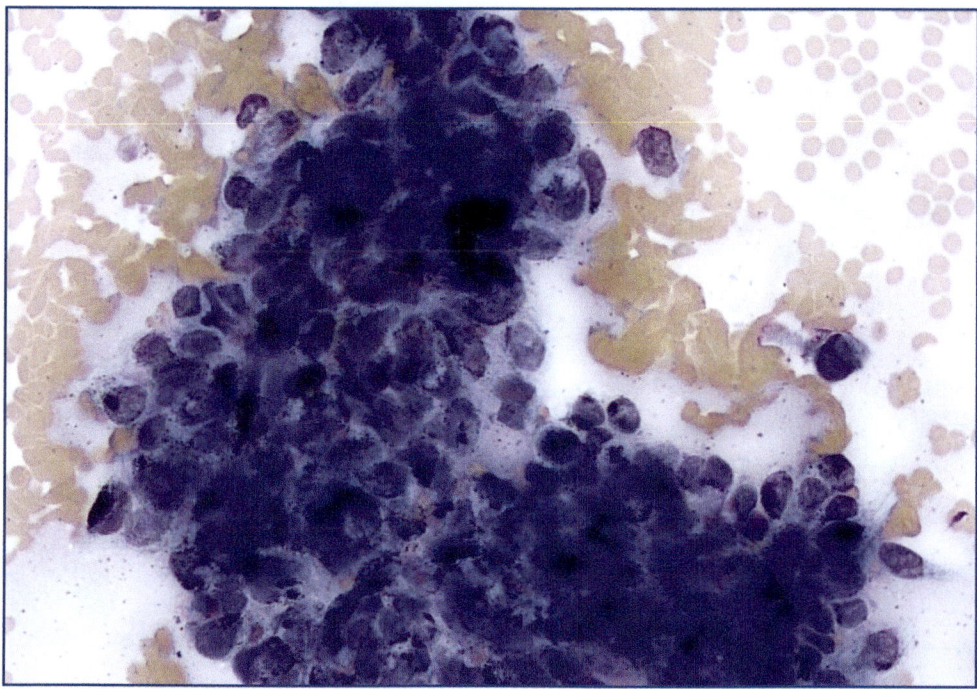

**Fig. 8.9.** Cat. Trichoblastoma. Tumour cells contain moderate amounts of black melanin pigment. Wright-Giemsa.

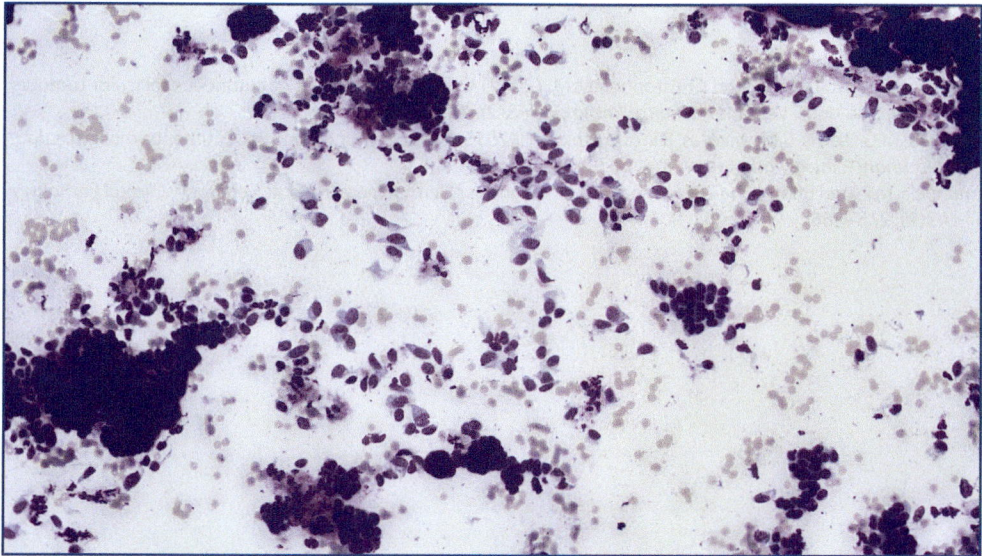

**Fig. 8.10.** Dog. Trichoblastoma. Numerous stromal cells are present amongst the neoplastic epithelial cells. Wright-Giemsa.

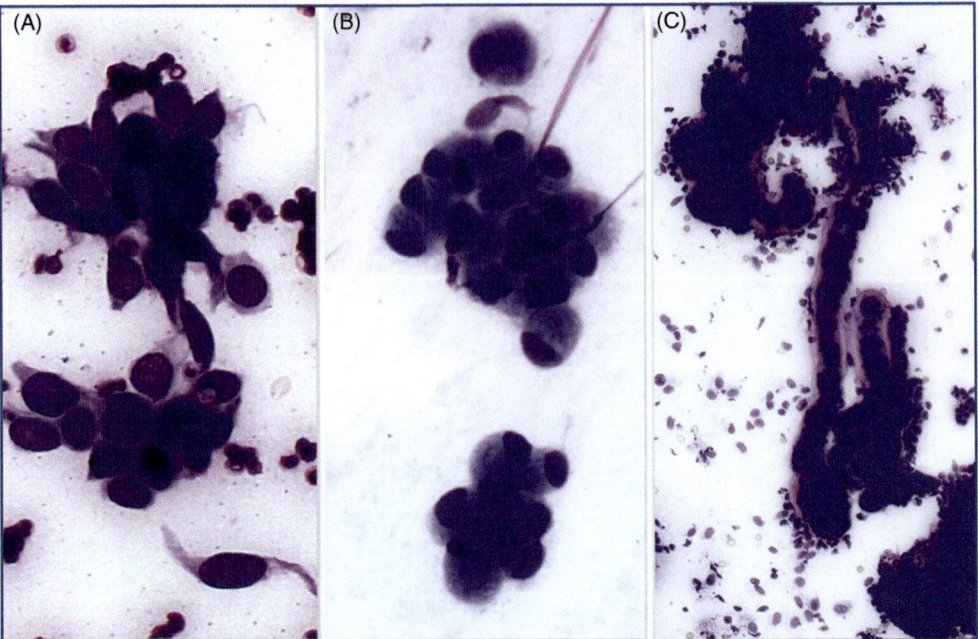

**Fig. 8.11.** Trichoblastoma variants: (A) Spindle cell variant. (B) Granular cell variant. (C) Ribbon/medusoid variant. Wright-Giemsa. *((A) and (B) courtesy of Tracy Stokol, Cornell University, USA.)*

## Further reading

Adedeji, A.O., Affolter, V.K. and Christopher, M.M. (2017) Cytological features of cutaneous follicular tumours and cysts in dogs. *Veterinary Clinical Pathology* 43(2), 143–150.

Asakawa, M.G., Lewis, S.M., Buckles, E.L. and Stokol, T. (2015) What is your diagnosis? Cutaneous mass in a dog. *Veterinary Clinical Pathology* 44(4), 607–608.

Emanuelli, M.P. and Bohn, A.A. (2014) What is your diagnosis? Dermal mass in a dog. *Veterinary Clinical Pathology* 43(2), 285–286.

# Trichoepithelioma

Follicular tumour that shows differentiation to all three segments of the hair follicle: *infundibulum, isthmus* and *inferior segment*.

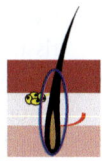

## Clinical features

- In dogs the overall incidence varies from 0.4% to 4% of all skin tumours. It is uncommon in cats, ranging from 0.3% to 0.8% of all skin tumours.
- Malignant trichoepithelioma is rare and is described only in dogs.
- Age:
  - Trichoepithelioma: peak of incidence between 5 and 11 years in dogs and 4 and 11 years in cats.
  - Malignant trichoepithelioma: between 8 and 12 years of age.
- Lesions can be single to multiple, round to ovoid or dome-shaped. Usually < 2 cm; larger masses (up to 15 cm) are less common. Malignant trichoepithelioma presents as a nodular infiltrative mass.
- It occurs more frequently on the dorsal trunk and legs but may affect other areas of the body.
- Trichoepithelioma carries a good prognosis. Malignant trichoepithelioma can metastasize to the draining lymph nodes and lungs.
- Over-represented canine breeds:
  - Trichoepithelioma: Basset Hound, Bullmastiff and Soft-coated Wheaten Terrier.
  - Malignant trichoepithelioma: Basset Hound and Airedale Terrier.

## Cytological features

- Cellularity is variable, from low to moderate.
- Background: usually lightly basophilic and granular with variable numbers of anucleated squamous epithelial cells. Cholesterol crystals and hair shafts may be present.
- Tumours are composed of epithelial islands and cystic structures containing keratinized squames. For this reason, aspirates may only yield sheets of keratin without nucleated cells.
- The cystic cavities contain anucleated squames and keratinized material, which can derive from all sections of the hair follicle. A mixture of the following structures is often observed cytologically:
  - Large polygonal corneocytes and/or liquid keratinized material: infundibulum.
  - Dense and homogeneous amorphous keratin: isthmus.
  - Ghost cells: inferior segment.
- Neoplastic cells are cuboidal (basaloid epithelial cells) and arranged in uniform cohesive clusters.
- Nuclei are small to medium sized with clumped chromatin and inconspicuous nucleoli.
- The cytoplasm is scant and pale basophilic.
- The N:C ratio is high and anisokaryosis and anisocytosis are minimal.

- Concurrent inflammation is common, especially if the keratin is exposed to the surrounding tissues. Mixed bacteria can also be seen.
- Malignant trichoepithelioma may show variable features of malignancy, such as hyperchromatic nuclei, increased anisokaryosis and anisocytosis and mitotic figures. Areas of necrosis may be present.

**Differential diagnoses**
- Follicular cyst (if no cuboidal epithelial cells are seen)
- Infundibular keratinizing achantoma
- Pilomatricoma (if only ghost cells are seen)
- Ductal adenoma of the sweat glands

**Pearls and Pitfalls**

In well-differentiated forms, the histological diagnosis of malignancy may be based only on the presence of infiltrative growth or vascular invasion, therefore cytology may be unable to recognize these lesions as malignant.

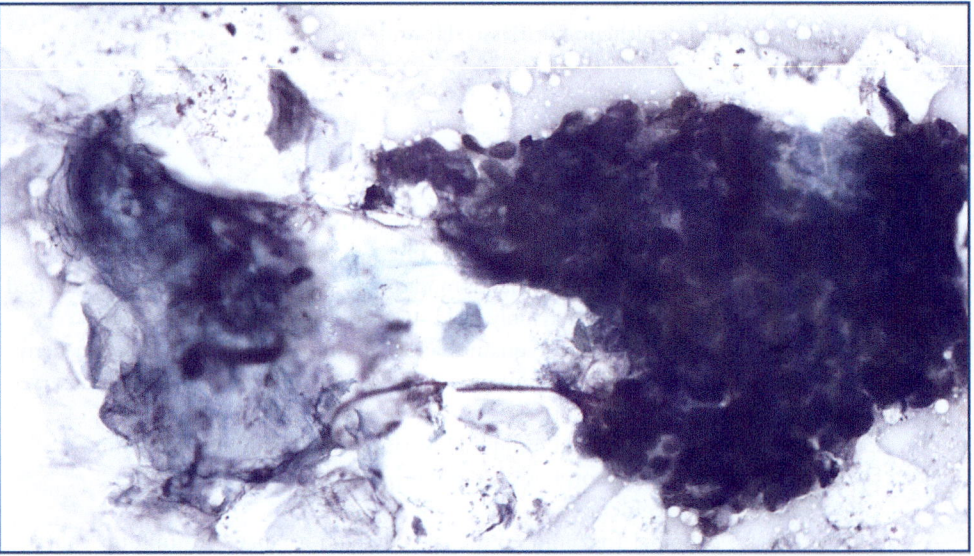

**Fig. 8.12.** Dog. Trichoepithelioma. There are cuboidal epithelial cells in dense cohesive clusters (right) and anucleated squamous epithelial cells (left). Wright-Giemsa.

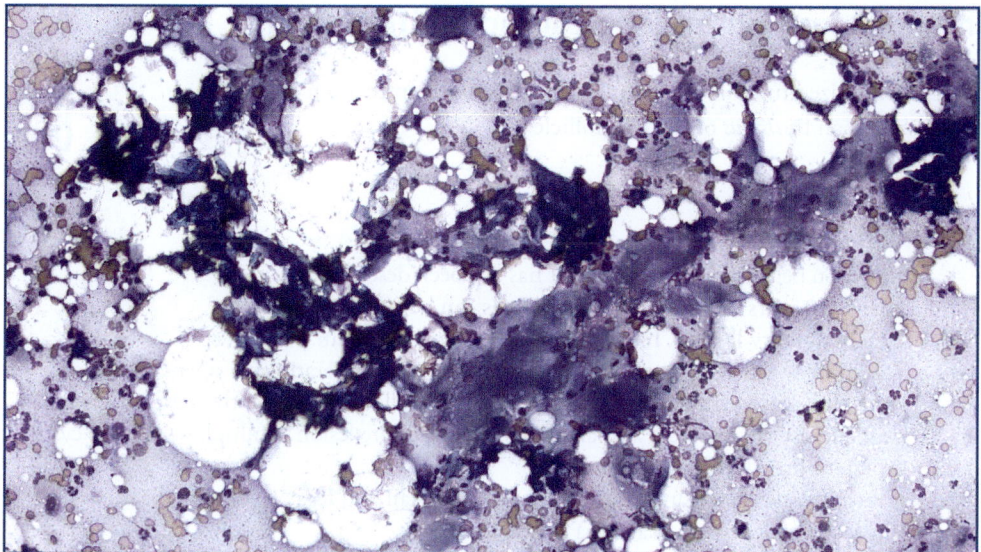

**Fig. 8.13.** Dog. Trichoepithelioma. There are numeorus anucleated squamous epithelial cells from the cystic area of the neoplasm. A concurrent neutrophilic inflammation is observed. Wright-Giemsa.

## Further reading

Adedeji, A.O., Affolter, V.K. and Christopher, M.M. (2017) Cytologic features of cutaneous follicular tumours and cysts in dogs. *Veterinary Clinical Pathology* 46(1), 143–150.

# Infundibular keratinizing acanthoma (IKA) (dog)

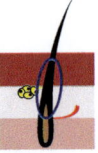

Benign keratinized tumour arising from the squamous epithelium of the *infundibulum* and *isthmus* of the hair follicle.

## Clinical features

- Common benign tumour in dogs. It has not been described in cats.
- Age: 4–10 years old, but younger animals can be affected.
- Usually solitary lesions, but multiple neoplasms can occur.
- This tumour generally has a large central cyst filled with keratin that opens on the surface of the skin with a central pore. The neoplastic cells are located at the periphery of the mass and usually represent a small portion of the entire lesion. Multiple secondary cystic lesions may develop over time.
- It most frequently occurs on the dorsum, neck, tail and legs.
- It is a benign lesion and carries a good prognosis.
- Over-represented canine breeds: Norwegian Elkhound, Tibetan Terrier, Pekingese.

## Cytological features

- Cellularity is variable.
- Background: lightly basophilic and variably haemodiluted.
- Fine-needle aspirates sampled from the large central cyst yielding a large amount of variably degenerating keratinized material, composed of polygonal anucleated squamous epithelial cells, amorphous keratin and cholesterol crystals. Nucleated neoplastic cells are often absent in the aspirates.
- If the needle is redirected in the areas composed of neoplastic cells, variable numbers of squamous epithelial cells at different maturation stages may be found.
- The nucleated cells, when present, may vary from basaloid epithelial cells to intermediate and mature squamous epithelial cells. An orderly progression throughout these stages can often be observed.
- A concurrent pyogranulomatous inflammation is common, especially when the wall of the cyst is compromised, leading to the exposure of the keratin to the surrounding tissues.

**Differential diagnoses**
- Follicular cyst (infundibular cyst and isthmus cyst)
- Trichoepithelioma

**Pearls and Pitfalls**

Ghost cells should not be found in aspirates from infundibular keratinizing acanthoma, as this tumour originates from the infundibulum and isthmus of the hair follicle only.

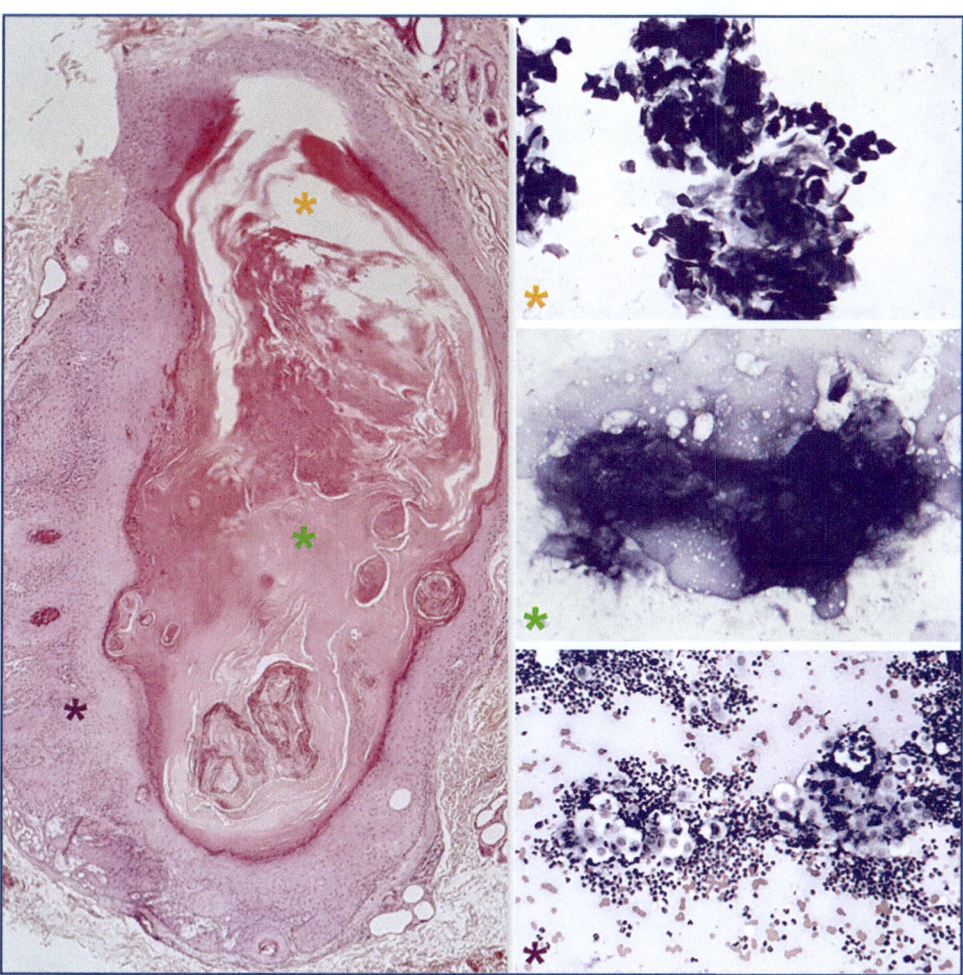

**Fig. 8.14.** Dog. IKA. Histopathological section (H&E) and cytological findings (Wright-Giemsa) from different areas of the tumour: the majority of the tumour area is occupied by a large cyst containing: *lamellar anucleated squamous epithelial cells in the superior segment (infundibulum) and *amorphous keratin in the lower part of the cyst (isthmus). *The tumour cells are confined to the outer part of the tumour. (*H&E section courtesy of Stefano Di Palma, Animal Health Trust, UK.*)

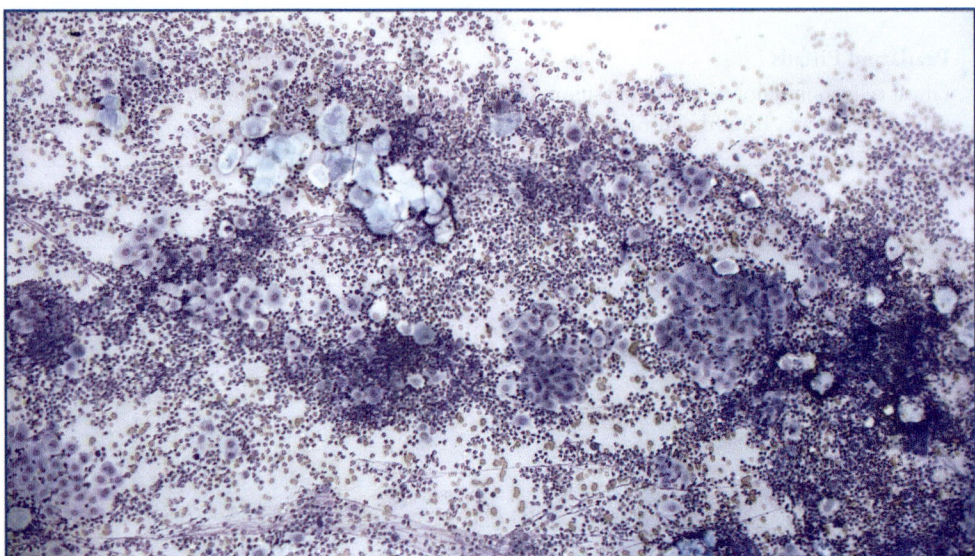

**Fig. 8.15.** Dog. IKA. There are moderate numbers of intermediate to mature squamous epithelial cells (tumour cells), lower numbers of anucleated squamous epithelial cells from the cystic area and numerous neutrophils. Wright-Giemsa.

# Pilomatricoma

Benign tumour that arises from the germinative cells of the follicular matrix or hair bulb.

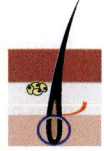

## Clinical features

- Uncommon benign tumour in dogs, accounting for approximately 3% of all skin epithelial neoplasms. The malignant counterpart is rare. Very rare in cats.
- Age in dogs: 2–7 years old.
- Lesions are usually solitary, firm and well circumscribed. Occasionally, multiple lesions can occur.
- Masses may have a gritty or bony consistency.
- It frequently occurs on legs, dorsal trunk, neck and tail.
- Most canine pilomatricomas are benign; malignant pilomatricoma is locally aggressive, with invasion and/or metastasis to the bone and metastasis to lymph nodes and lung.
- Over-represented canine breeds: Standard Poodle, Kerry Blue Terrier, Old English Sheepdog, Soft-coated Wheaten Terrier, Airedale Terrier, Bouvier des Flandres, Bichon Frise, Schnauzer and Basset Hound.

## Cytological features

- Aspirates usually yield a large amount of specimen, with or without low numbers of intact nucleated cells.
- Characterized by high numbers of ghost cells. These are anucleated squamous epithelial cells with a pale central area. They are polygonal, often hexagonal, and relatively small compared with the polygonal anucleated squamous epithelial cells from the infundibulum.
- Occasionally, small clusters of uniform cuboidal epithelial cells may be found.
- Secondary inflammation is possible, especially if the keratin is exposed to the surrounding tissues.
- Malignant pilomatricoma may be well differentiated and may not differ morphologically from a benign pilomatricoma. Occasionally, variable features of malignancy, such as slightly disorganized clusters, increased anisokaryosis and anisocytosis and mitotic figures may be observed. Areas of necrosis may be present.

**Differential diagnosis**

Follicular cyst (matrical cyst)

**Pearls and Pitfalls**

Malignant pilomatricoma may lack morphological features of atypia and the histological diagnosis of malignancy is often based only on the presence of infiltration of the surrounding tissues and vascular invasion.

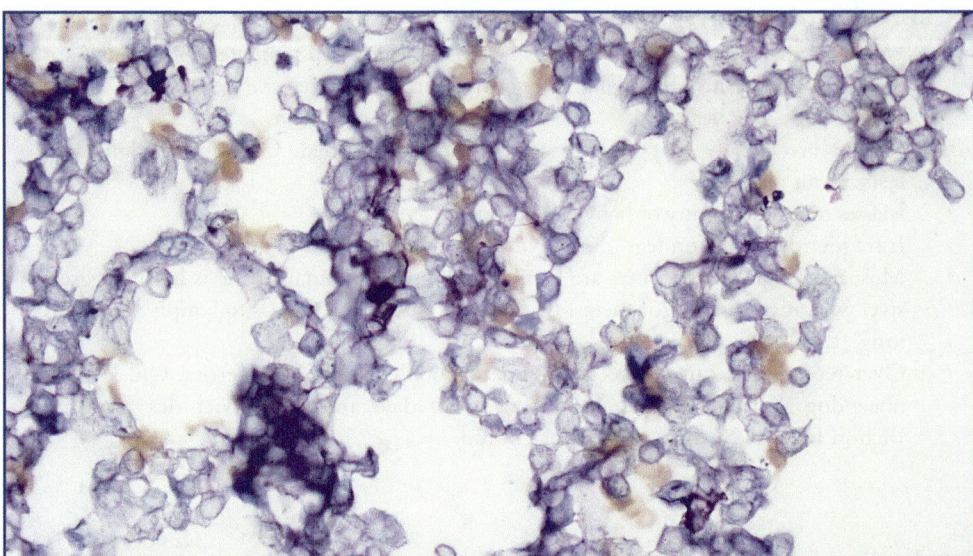

**Fig. 8.16.** Dog. Pilomatricoma. Numerous ghost cells seen. Another cytological differential for these findings is a matrical cyst. Wright-Giemsa.

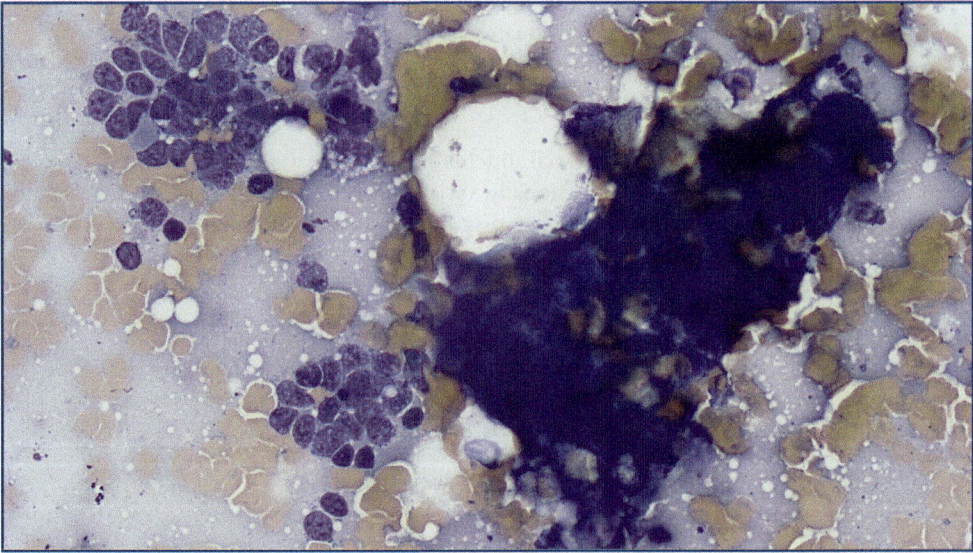

**Fig. 8.17.** Dog. Malignant pilomatricoma. Cuboidal epithelial cells lacking significant criteria or malignancy. The diagnosis of malignancy was achieved on histopathology. Wright-Giemsa.

# Further reading

Carroll, E.E., Fossey, S.L., Mangus, L.M., Carsillo, M.E., Rush, L.J., McLeod, C.G. and Johnson, T.O. (2010) Malignant pilomatricoma in 3 dogs. *Veterinary Pathology* 47(5), 937–943.

Jackson, K., Boger, L., Goldschmidt, M. and Walton, R.M. (2010) Malignant pilomatricoma in a soft-coated Wheaten Terrier. *Veterinary Clinical Pathology* 39(2), 236–240.

Masserdotti, C. and Ubbiali, F.A. (2002) Fine needle aspiration cytology of pilomatricoma in three dogs. *Veterinary Clinical Pathology* 31(1), 22–25.

## 8.4 Sebaceous Tumours

### Sebaceous adenoma, epithelioma and carcinoma

Tumours that arise from the sebaceous epithelial cells in the dermis.

### Clinical features

- Sebaceous adenoma:
    - Common benign tumour of dogs and rare in cats, except for Persian cats.
    - Age in dogs: 8–13 years old.
    - Lesions are usually solitary, often exophytic (pedunculated). They can be alopecic, hyperpigmented and ulcerated.
    - In dogs, it more frequently occurs on the head.
    - In cats, it arises most commonly on the head, tail and back.
    - Over-represented canine breeds: Cocker Spaniel, Siberian Husky.
- Sebaceous epithelioma:
    - Common tumour in dogs and rare in cats.
    - Age in dogs: 10–15 years old.
    - It most commonly arises on the head.
    - It can appear macroscopically dark/black, as the tumour may contain melanocytes.
    - Over-represented canine breeds: Irish Water Spaniel, Cocker Spaniel, German Wirehaired Pointer and Canadian Eskimo Dog.
- Sebaceous carcinoma:
    - Rare tumour in both dogs and cats.
    - Age: 10–13 years old in dogs; 8–15 years old in cats.
    - Lesions are usually solitary, multilobulated, often alopecic and ulcerated.
    - In dogs, it more frequently occurs on the head and neck.
    - In cats, it more commonly arises on the head, thorax and perineum.
    - Metastasis to the draining lymph nodes can occur.
    - Over-represented canine breeds: Cavalier King Charles Spaniel, Cocker Spaniel, Siberian Husky, Samoyed and West Highland White Terrier.

### Cytological features

- Cellularity is variable, generally moderate.
- Background: clear or pale basophilic. It occasionally contains a variable amount of negatively staining amorphous material (sebum).
- Sebaceous adenoma:
    - The tumour is composed of a predominance of sebocytes with low numbers of reserve cells and ducts.
    - Sebocytes are well differentiated and arranged in variably sized, often tridimensional clusters.
    - Nuclei are small, dense and central.
    - The cytoplasm is abundant and heavily vacuolated. It contains numerous small, clear, punctate vacuoles.
    - Anisokaryosis and anisocytosis are minimal. The N:C ratio is low.
    - Low numbers of reserve epithelial cells may be seen (less than 50% of the cells). These are uniform cuboidal epithelial cells with small round nuclei and scant cytoplasm.

- Sebaceous epithelioma:
  - The tumour is composed of a predominance of reserve cells with a few sebocytes and ducts.
  - The aspirates often yield relatively large cohesive clusters of cuboidal reserve epithelial cells admixed with small clusters of mature sebocytes. The reserve epithelial cells often outnumber the mature sebaceous epithelial cells.
  - Nuclei are small, dense and central, often with inconspicuous nucleoli.
  - The cytoplasm is scant and pale to moderately basophilic. It occasionally contains low numbers of variably sized (but often small) clear vacuoles.
  - Anisokaryosis and anisocytosis are minimal. The N:C ratio is high.
- Sebaceous carcinoma:
  - Cellularity is variable, usually high.
  - Background: lightly to moderately basophilic and finely granular. It can contain variably sized punctate clear vacuoles.
  - The aspirates are composed of variably sized, cohesive clusters of cuboidal epithelial cells. Admixed with these cells, there might be low numbers of well-differentiated sebocytes.
  - Nuclei are round, medium-large and with a finely stippled chromatin. Nucleoli are variably visible.
  - The cytoplasm is scant to moderate and moderately basophilic. It can contain variably sized clear vacuoles.
  - Anisokaryosis, anisocytosis and degree of pleomorphism are variable.
  - Cell crowding is frequent. Nuclear moulding is occasionally observed.
  - Mitotic figures can be found.

---

**Differential diagnoses**
- Sebaceous adenoma:
  - Sebaceous hyperplasia
  - Fibroadnexal hamartoma
- Sebaceous epithelioma and carcinoma:
  - Liposarcoma
  - Clear cell adnexal carcinoma

**Pearls and Pitfalls**

- A less common benign adenoma arising from the sebaceous glands is the sebaceous duct adenoma. This is composed of a predominance of ducts (>50%) with a smaller proportion of secretory sebocytes and reserve cells. The ducts often contain keratin and occasionally sebum. Upon aspiration, these may exfoliate variable numbers of anucleated squamous epithelial cells, sebocytes and cuboidal to columnar ductal cells.
- Cytologically, sebaceous adenoma cannot be distinguished from nodular sebaceous hyperplasia. This does not have any clinical implication, as they are both benign lesions that carry a good prognosis.
- The cytological differentiation between sebaceous epithelioma and a well-differentiated sebaceous carcinoma can be very challenging. However, whilst epithelioma is relatively common, sebaceous carcinoma is a rare tumour.
- On the eyelids, there are modified sebaceous glands called Meibomian glands. Adenomas arising from the Meibomian glands are cytologically similar to the classical sebaceous adenomas described above.

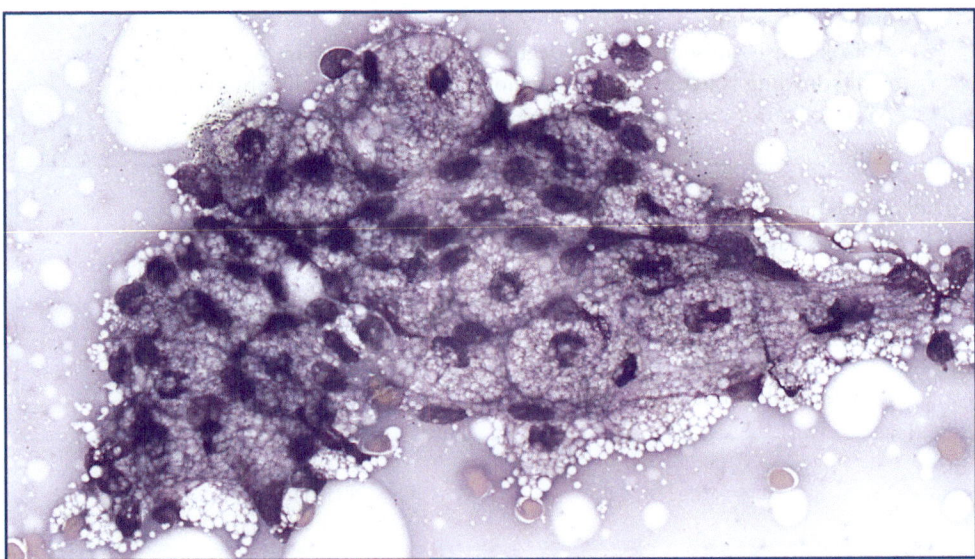

**Fig. 8.18.** Dog. Sebaceous adenoma. Mature sebocytes arranged in a cohesive cluster. Wright-Giemsa.

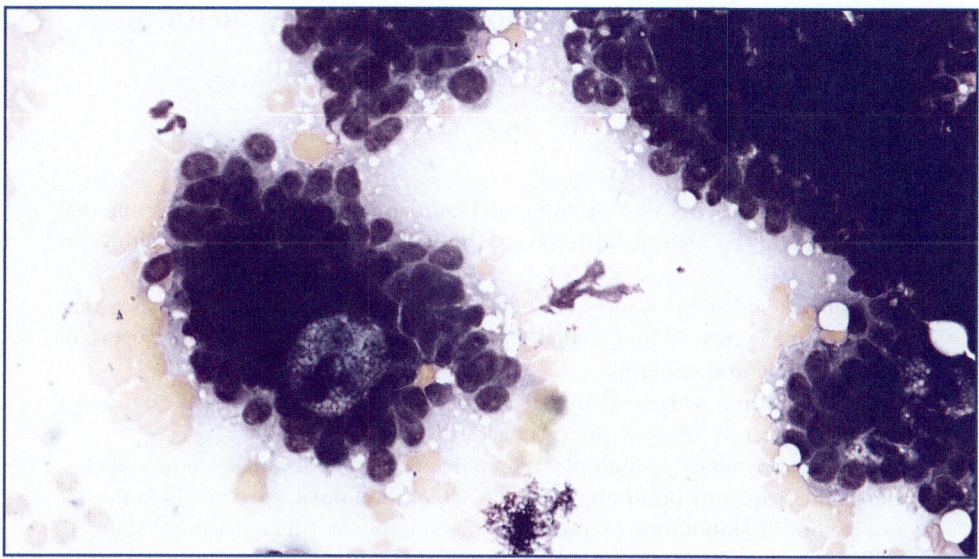

**Fig. 8.19.** Dog. Sebaceous epithelioma. Reserve epithelial cells outnumber the mature sebocytes. Wright-Giemsa.

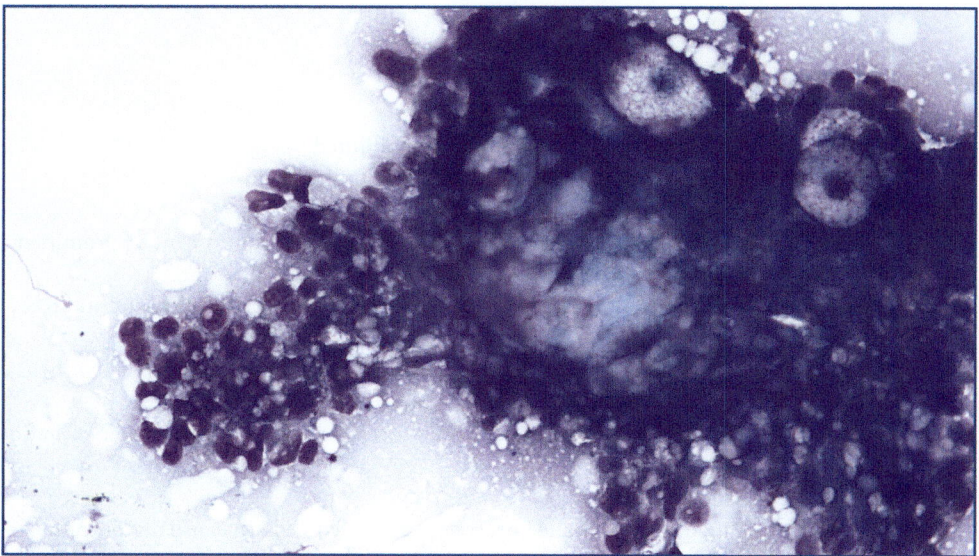

**Fig. 8.20.** Dog. Sebaceous carcinoma. Clusters of cuboidal epithelial cells admixed with low numbers of mature sebocytes. Cuboidal cells display an irregular vacuolation. Criteria of malignancy are mild. Wright-Giemsa.

# Perianal gland adenoma, epithelioma and carcinoma (dog)

Tumours arising from hepatoid glands, which are modified sebaceous glands.

## Clinical features

- Perianal gland tumours are very common (approximately 18% of all skin tumours).
- Three types of perianal gland tumours are described: adenoma, epithelioma and carcinoma.
- Perianal gland adenoma is more frequent than epithelioma. Carcinoma is very rare.
- Age: 8–9 to 13 years old for perianal gland adenoma and epithelioma; 6–15 years old for perianal gland carcinoma.
- Sex predisposition: perianal gland adenoma is androgen related and male entire dogs are most frequently affected. Intact females are at lower risk.
- Lesions can be solitary or multiple, exophytic or endophytic and often ulcerated.
- They more frequently occur on the caudal half of the animal, particularly in the perianal region, tail, hindlimbs, prepuce area, mammary areas (in female dogs) and in the midline of thorax and dorsum.
- In perianal gland adenoma, castration may reduce the size of the mass. Perianal gland carcinoma may occasionally metastasize to the regional lymph nodes.
- Perianal gland epithelioma is regarded as a low-grade malignancy.

## Cytological features

- Cellularity is variable, often moderate to high.
- Background: clear or pale basophilic and often haemodiluted.
- Neoplastic cells exfoliate in medium-large cohesive and uniform clusters.
- Perianal gland adenoma:
    - Nuclei are medium sized with a reticular chromatin and a round central prominent nucleolus. Occasionally two to three nucleoli are seen.
    - The cytoplasm is abundant, lightly to moderately amphophilic to basophilic and has a fine grainy texture.
    - Low numbers of reserve epithelial cells may be seen. They are small cuboidal epithelial cells with small, round nuclei and scant cytoplasm.
    - Anisokaryosis is mild and anisocytosis is mild, occasionally moderate. The N:C ratio is low.
- Perianal gland epithelioma:
    - Aspirates exfoliate a predominance of reserve epithelial cells that usually outnumber the mature component.
    - Nuclei are small to medium sized, round and have dense chromatin and inconspicuous nucleoli.
    - The cytoplasm is scant and pale to moderately basophilic.
    - Anisokaryosis and anisocytosis are minimal.
- Perianal gland carcinoma:
    - Neoplastic cells are usually still relatively well differentiated but may be in more disorganized clusters. Cellular pleomorphism may occasionally be more prominent and nuclei may contain multiple prominent, occasionally angular and variably sized nucleoli. The N:C ratio might be reduced.

- Rarely, mature sebocytes may be seen amongst the modified perianal gland epithelial cells, in both adenomas and carcinomas. These cells are heavily vacuolated.
- In some tumours, squamous metaplasia of the ductal epithelial cells can occur. In these cases, variable numbers of anucleated squamous epithelial cells and occasionally cholesterol crystals may be seen.

**Differential diagnoses**
- Perianal gland adenoma:
    - Well-differentiated perianal gland carcinoma
    - Perianal gland epithelioma
- Perianal gland carcinoma:
    - Perianal gland adenoma
    - Perianal gland epithelioma

**Pearls and Pitfalls**
- Perianal gland carcinoma does not always show significant cytological features of atypia and may exfoliate well-differentiated hepatoid cells. Due to this, a more general diagnosis of perianal gland tumour might be preferred, with the specification that adenoma is common and carcinoma is rare.
- A single case report of a squamous cell carcinoma arising within a perianal gland adenoma was described in a dog. Cytology was characterized by well-differentiated perianal gland epithelial cells and anucleated squamous epithelial cells. No atypical squamous epithelial cells exfoliated upon aspiration.

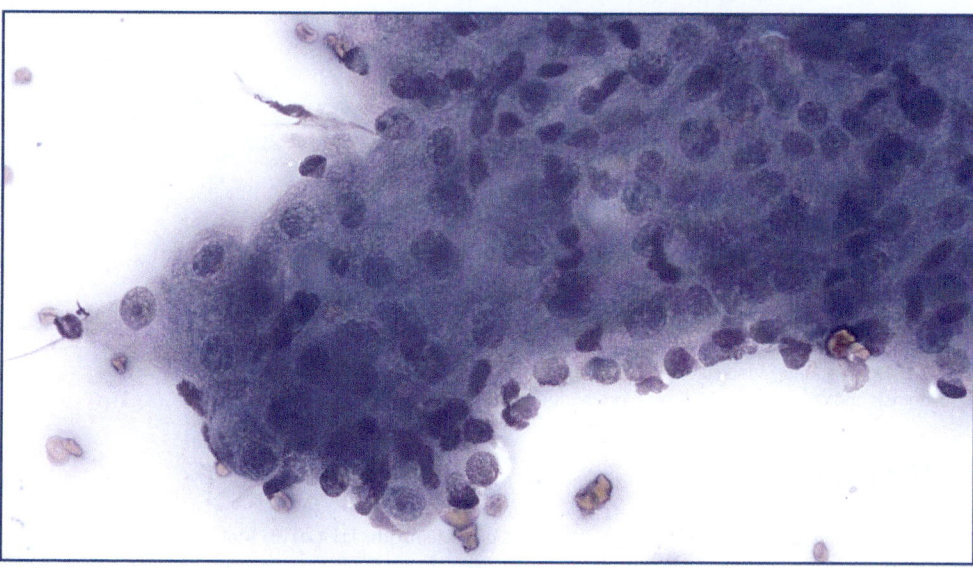

**Fig. 8.21.** Dog. Perianal gland adenoma. Mature hepatoid gland cells in a cohesive uniform cluster. Wright-Giemsa.

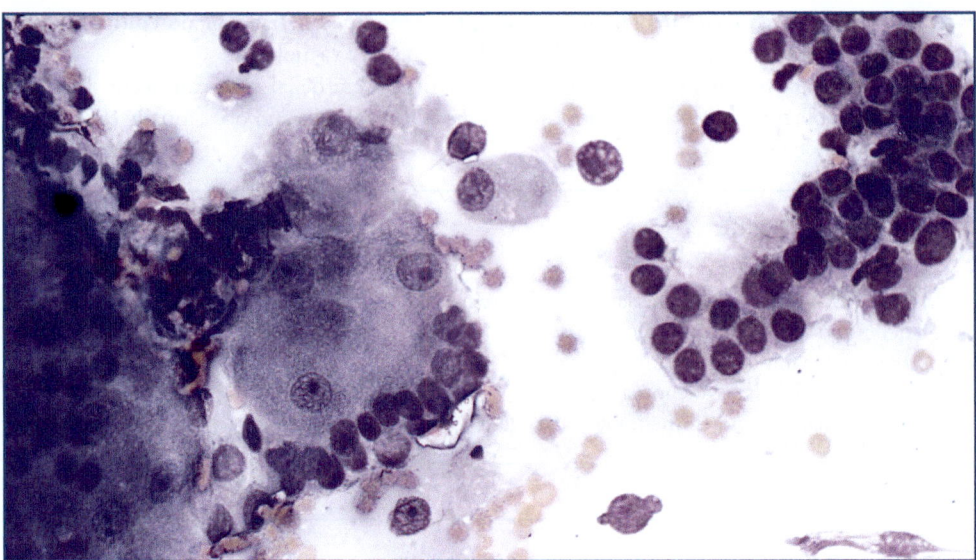

**Fig. 8.22.** Dog. Perianal gland epithelioma. Reserve epithelial cells are numerous and outnumber the mature hepatoid gland cells. Wright-Giemsa.

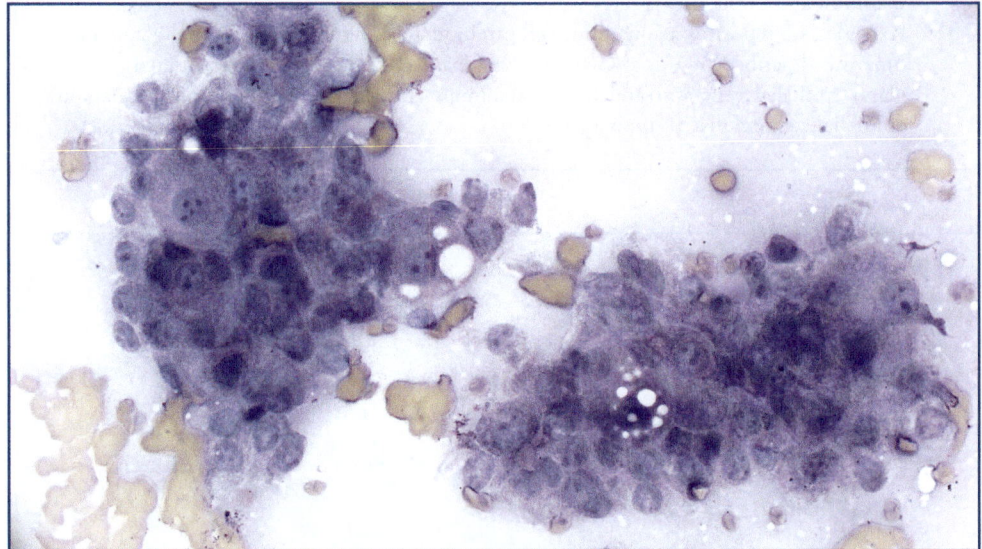

**Fig. 8.23.** Dog. Perianal gland carcinoma. Hepatoid gland cells are moderately pleomorphic and display moderate anisokaryosis and anisocytosis. Multiple prominent nucleoli are present. Wright-Giemsa.

## Further reading

McCourt, M.R., Levine, G.M., Breshears, M.A., Wall, C.R. and Meinkoth, J.H. (2018) Metastatic disease in a dog with a well-differentiated perianal gland tumor. *Veterinary Clinical Pathology*, early view, 10.1111/vcp.12662.

Stewart, J. and Monti, P. (2015) What is your diagnosis? Perianal mass in a dog. *Veterinary Clinical Pathology* 44, 615–616.

# 8.5 Apocrine Gland Tumours

## Sweat gland adenoma and carcinoma

Tumours arising from the apocrine and eccrine glands.

### Clinical features
- Apocrine adenoma and apocrine duct adenoma:
    - Common in both dogs and cats.
    - Age: adult animals are more frequently affected.
    - Apocrine adenoma and apocrine duct adenoma usually occur on the head and neck in both dogs and cats. Other locations for apocrine duct adenoma in dogs are neck, thorax and legs.
    - Tumours can be localized in the dermis or subcutis and can be multilobulated and cystic. They feel soft on palpation. Apocrine tumours with a cystic cavity often have a bluish colour due to the dark tint of the cystic fluid.
    - There is no breed predisposition for apocrine adenoma in dogs and cats.
    - Over-represented breeds for apocrine duct adenoma:
        - Dogs: Tibetan Terrier, Old English Sheepdog, Pyrenean Mountain Dog, Bernese Mountain Dog and Golden Retriever.
        - Cats: Persian and Himalayan cats.
- Apocrine carcinoma and apocrine duct carcinoma:
    - Apocrine carcinoma is relatively common in dogs, less so in cats. Apocrine duct carcinoma is rare in both species.
    - Apocrine carcinoma usually occurs on the head, axillary and inguinal areas in both dogs and cats.
    - Tumours can be in the dermis or subcutis. Inflammation and ulceration are possible.
    - Over-represented breeds for apocrine carcinoma and duct carcinoma:
        - Dogs: Norwegian Elkhound, Chow Chow, Newfoundland, Shi Tzu, Old English Sheepdog, Australian Shepherd, Keeshond.
        - Cats: Siamese cats.
- Eccrine adenoma and carcinoma:
    - These tumours originate from the eccrine glands and, in dogs and cats, are confined to the footpads. These tumours are very rare in both species.

### Cytological features
- Apocrine adenoma and apocrine duct adenoma:
    - They share similar cytological characteristics, though in duct adenomas columnar cells are more frequently found.
    - Cellularity is often low to moderate. If the aspirates are from the cystic area of the tumour, the preparations might be acellular or only contain rare foamy macrophages and scattered cholesterol crystals.
    - Background: clear or pale basophilic and variably haemodiluted.

- Apocrine cells are cuboidal to columnar and exfoliate in small cohesive and uniform clusters.
- Nuclei are small, round, with finely stippled chromatin. Nucleoli are usually inconspicuous.
- The cytoplasm is scant, occasionally moderate and pale basophilic. It can contain small, dark granules of secretory product.
- Anisokaryosis and anisocytosis are minimal and the N:C ratio is moderate to high.
- Apocrine carcinoma and apocrine duct carcinoma:
  - They share similar cytological findings.
  - Cellularity is variable, usually high.
  - Cells are cuboidal to columnar and exfoliate in medium-large cohesive clusters. Clusters may be disorganized and cells may show nuclear moulding and crowding.
  - Nuclei are generally medium sized, round and with finely stippled chromatin. Nucleoli can be variably visible, from indistinct to prominent, single or multiple.
  - The cytoplasm is scant and pale to moderately basophilic and may contain dark granules.
  - Anisokaryosis and anisocytosis are variable and may be marked. The N:C ratio is moderate to high.
- Eccrine adenoma and carcinoma:
  - Cytologically they mirror the apocrine adenoma and carcinoma.

---

**Differential diagnoses**

- Apocrine adenoma and duct adenoma:
  - Trichoblastoma
  - Basal cell tumour
  - Mammary adenoma (depending on the location of the mass)
- Apocrine carcinoma and duct carcinoma:
  - Mammary carcinoma (depending on the location of the mass)
- Eccrine carcinoma:
  - Metastatic pulmonary carcinoma in cats (due to the location of the lesions in the footpads)

---

**Pearls and Pitfalls**

- Apocrine and duct apocrine adenomas are very similar cytologically. For this reason a more broad diagnosis of sweat gland adenoma can be made. The distinction between these two forms does not have any clinical implication, as they are both benign and respond well to surgical excision.
- Both adenoma and carcinoma (secretory or ductal) can have areas of squamous differentiation. This may result in the presence of anucleated squamous epithelial cells in the aspirates, alongside the glandular epithelial cells.
- As for mammary tumours, complex and mixed adenoma and carcinoma of the sweat glands have been described. In complex adenoma and carcinoma, alongside the epithelial component, myoepithelial cells are observed. In mixed sweat gland adenoma and carcinoma, a cartilaginous and/or osseous metaplasia of the myoepithelial cells is found. These are rare tumours in dogs and cats.

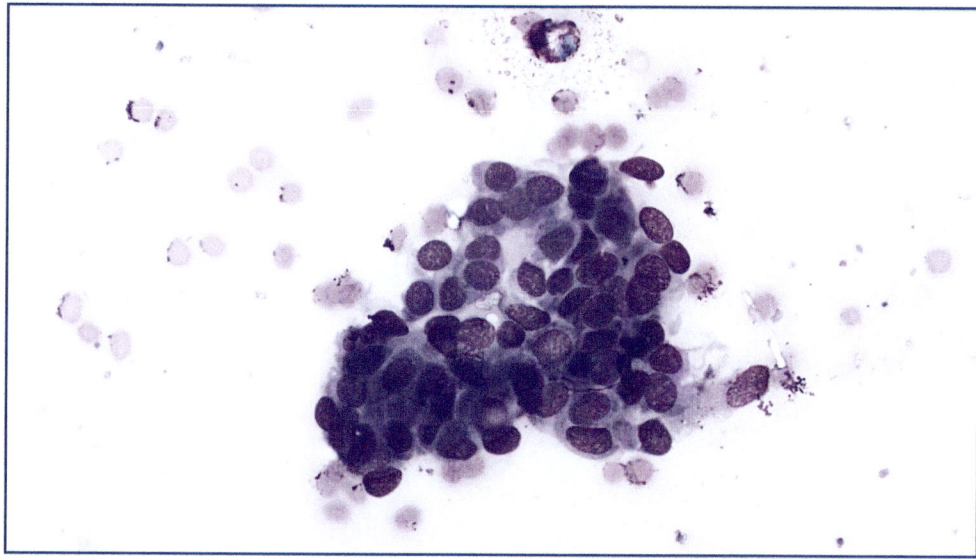

**Fig. 8.24.** Dog. Sweat gland adenoma. Cluster of uniform columnar epithelial cells. Wright-Giemsa.

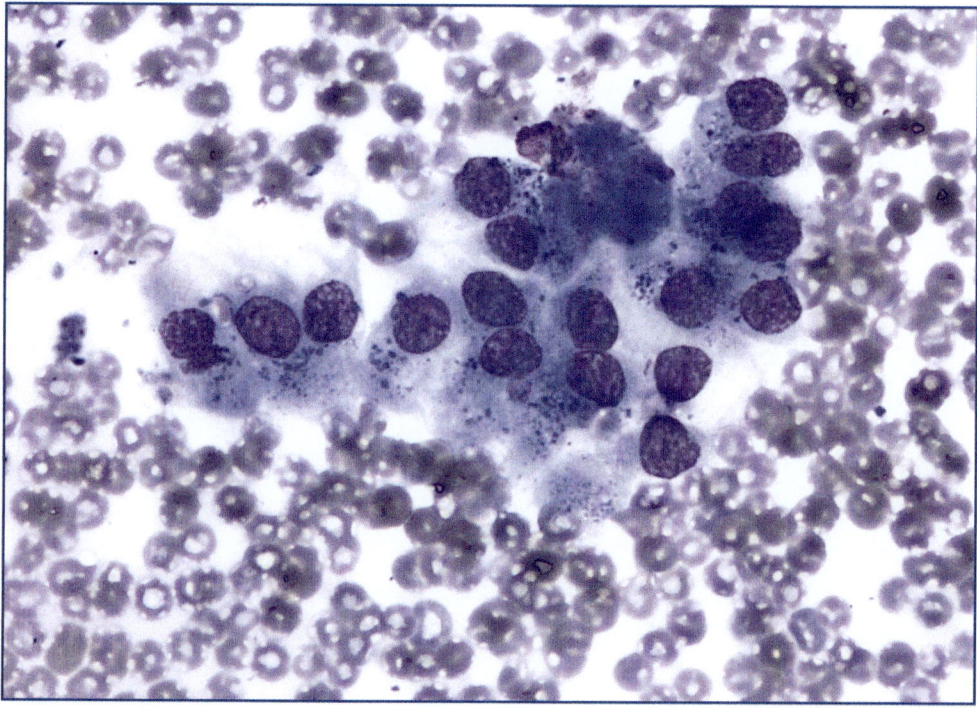

**Fig. 8.25.** Cat. Sweat gland adenoma. Apocrine columnar epithelial cells with intracytoplasmatic granules of secretory material. Wright-Giemsa.

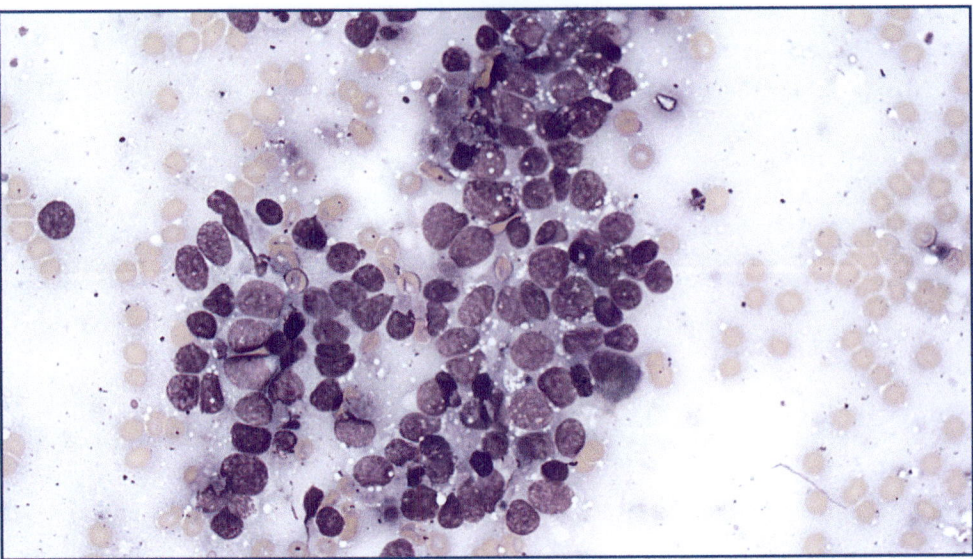

**Fig. 8.26.** Dog. Sweat gland carcinoma. Cuboidal epithelial cells arranged in a moderately disorganized cluster. Cells display moderate anisokaryosis and occasionally contain poorly visible nucleoli. Wright-Giemsa.

# Ceruminous gland adenoma and carcinoma

Tumours arising from the specialized sweat glands of the ear canal.

## Clinical features
- Ceruminous gland adenoma:
  - Common in both dogs and cats.
  - Age: the peak incidence is between 7 and 10 years of age in both species.
  - Usually exophytic masses within the external ear canal.
  - They can be ulcerated and infected.
  - Over-represented canine breeds: Cocker Spaniel, Shih Tzu, Toy Poodle, Pekingese.
- Ceruminous gland carcinoma:
  - More common in cats than in dogs.
  - Age: the peak incidence in cats is between 7 and 13 years of age; in dogs between 10 and 12 years of age.
  - Often presents as an infiltrative, erosive and ulcerated mass in the external ear canal.
  - Over-represented feline breeds: Domestic Short Hair
  - Over-represented canine breeds: Bull Terrier, Shih Tzu, Cocker Spaniel, Belgian Shepherd Dog (Malinois).

## Cytological features
- Cellularity is variable.
- Background: pale basophilic, variably haemodiluted. It can contain black–blue granular material and amorphous extracellular material corresponding to cerumen (earwax).
- Cells exfoliate in variably sized cohesive clusters. They are cuboidal, columnar or polygonal and have a variable N:C ratio.
- Nuclei are round, small to medium sized in adenomas; larger and more pleomorphic in carcinomas. One or multiple prominent nucleoli can be seen in carcinomas.
- The cytoplasm is usually moderate in amount and pale to moderately basophilic. It sometimes contains small black to dark green granules of secretory material.
- Mixed inflammatory cells can be found, especially if the tumour is ulcerated. These include neutrophils and macrophages, which may contain amorphous phagosomes.
- Mitoses can be seen in carcinomas.

**Pearls and Pitfalls**

Clinical differential diagnoses for these tumours include:

- Cats: inflammatory polyps arising from the middle ear and extending to the external ear canal. Upon aspiration, inflammatory polyps may exfoliate either large polygonal or oval epithelial cells arranged singly or in small clusters and/or cells with respiratory epithelial differentiation. The latter are columnar with round, basal nuclei and a moderate amount of light basophilic cytoplasm, sometimes with apical cilia. Cells may contain small granules of secretory material. Concurrent inflammation is common.

- Dogs: hyperplastic polypoid otitis externa.

- The diagnosis of well-differentiated carcinoma lacking significant pleomorphism is made on histopathology when invasion of the adjacent tissues and numbers of mitoses are observed.

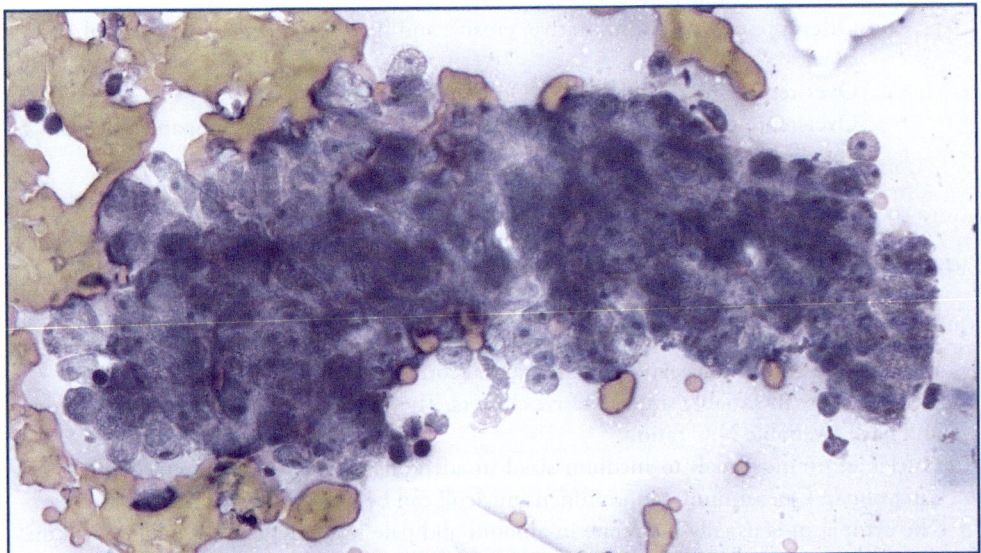

**Fig. 8.27.** Cat. Ceruminous gland carcinoma. Mildly disorganized clusters of ceruminous epithelial cells. They display crowding and have a high N:C ratio. Nuclei have a coarse chromatin and one to multiple prominent nucleoli. Wright-Giemsa.

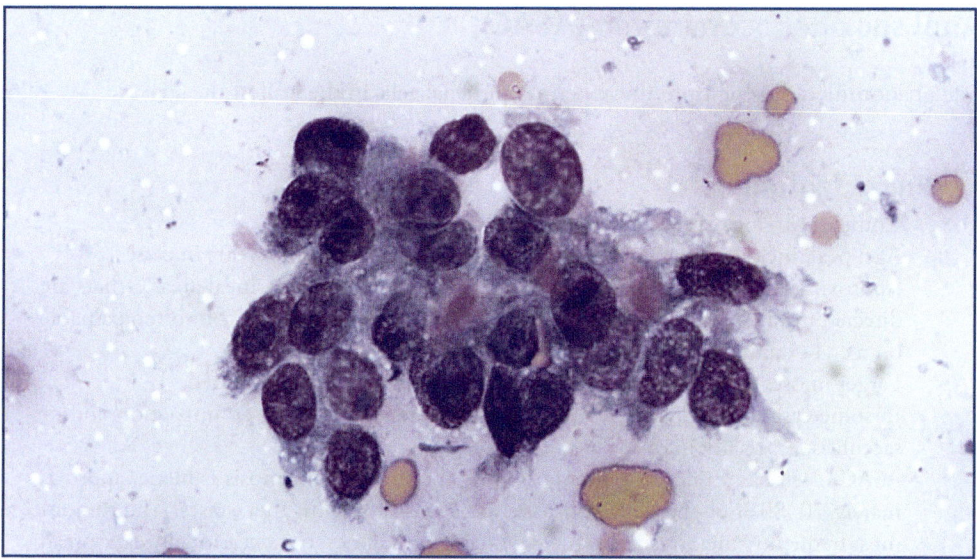

**Fig. 8.28.** Cat. Ceruminous gland carcinoma. Cells are more differentiated compared with the example above. They are columnar and display mild to moderate anisokaryosis. A central prominent nucleolus is present. Wright-Giemsa.

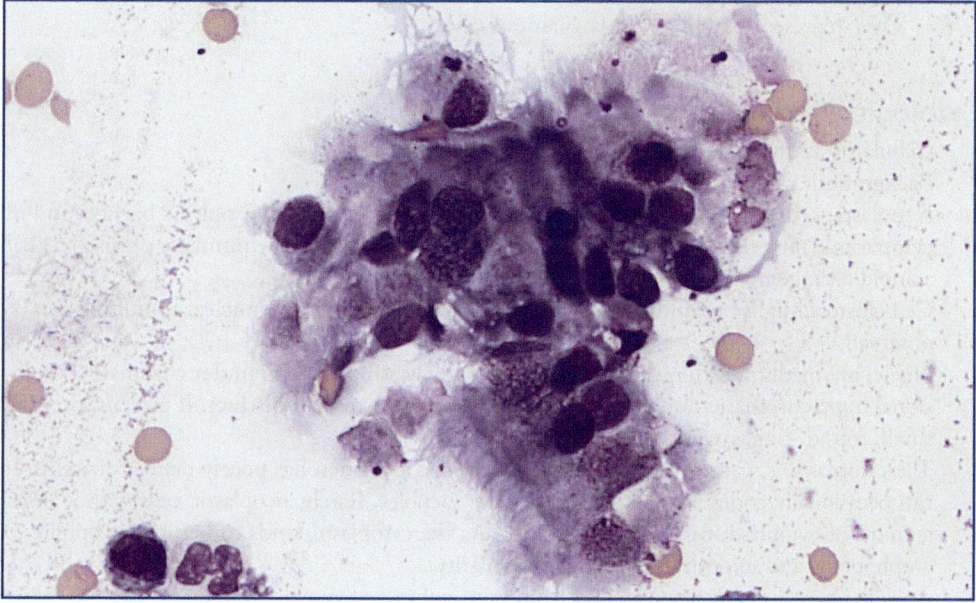

**Fig. 8.29.** Cat. Ear polyp. Ciliated columnar epithelial cells (respiratory differentiation). Wright-Giemsa.

# Further reading

De Lorenzi, D., Bonfanti, U., Masserdotti, C. and Tranquillo, M. (2005) Fine-needle biopsy of external ear canal masses in the cat: cytologic results and histologic correlations in 27 cases. *Veterinary Clinical Pathology* 34(2), 100–105.

# Anal sac adenocarcinoma (ASAC)

Malignant tumour arising from the apocrine epithelial cells in the wall of the anal sac.

## Clinical features
- Common in dogs and rare in cats.
- Age: peak incidence between 8 and 12 years in dogs and 6–17 years in cats.
- Approximately half of the tumours present as masses in the perineal area. Others are directed inwards, and masses may not be visible from the outside, but often palpable on rectal examination.
- Larger masses can cause difficulties in defecation and can be ulcerated.
- In some cases, ASAC can present with signs referable to anal sac impaction and/or sacculitis, especially in cats.
- ASAC often has an occult presentation. By the time the diagnosis is made, approximately 70–80% of the dogs will have local and/or distant metastases. The tumour most frequently metastasizes to the regional lymph nodes, but occasionally can spread to other organs, in particular lung, liver, spleen and bone.
- In cats, the presumptive metastatic rate is approximately 16%.
- Over-represented canine breeds: Cocker Spaniel, English Springer Spaniel, Cavalier King Charles Spaniel, Dandie Dinmont Terrier, German Shepherd Dog.
- Over-represented feline breeds: Siamese cat.

## Cytological features
- Cellularity is often moderate to high.
- Background: variably haemodiluted and pale basophilic.
- Neoplastic cells can present as naked nuclei embedded in a pale basophilic background of cytoplasmic material or as intact cells in cohesive clusters. Variable numbers of rosette-like/ acinoid arrangements are seen.
- Cell clusters might be mildly disorganized and cell crowding and nuclear moulding can be observed.
- Nuclei are medium to large, round, and have finely stippled to granular chromatin. Occasional hyperchromatic nuclei can be present. Nucleoli can be indistinct. If present, they are small, round, single or multiple.
- The cytoplasm is scant to moderate, pale basophilic and often has poorly defined margins. It can occasionally contain small, clear, punctate vacuoles. Rarely, neoplastic cells with a larger amount of cytoplasm can be seen. In this case, the cytoplasm tends to be pale basophilic to amphophilic and smooth (without any granularity).
- Anisokaryosis and anisocytosis vary from minimal to occasionally moderate. The N:C ratio is high. Mitoses can occasionally be observed.
- Low to moderate numbers of inflammatory cells can be present, including activated macrophages and granulated mast cells.
- The aspirates can occasionally contain variable numbers of anucleated squamous epithelial cells and extracellular bacteria, which suggest concurrent anal sac impaction.

**Pearls and Pitfalls**
- Cellular atypia is often minimal giving the tumour a 'benign' appearance, in spite of its aggressive clinical behaviour.
- In dogs, ASAC can be associated with a paraneoplastic hypercalcaemia. These patients often develop polyuria and polydipsia.

## Variants

There are multiple histological variants, which represent different degrees of differentiation of the tumour. Common variants include the solid, rosette and tubular types. Less common are the clear cell and signet ring variants. In a recent study, the solid growth pattern was shown to have a significantly poorer outcome.

**Differential diagnoses**
- Canine clitoral carcinoma (different localization)
- Sweat gland adenoma or carcinoma arising in skin in the perineal area

**Pearls and Pitfalls**

A rare morphological variant (atypical or spindle cell variant) is described cytologically and histologically. This form is characterized by a large proportion of polygonal to elongated neoplastic cells, occasionally forming rosette-like patterns. Nuclei are round to oval and have fine, uniform chromatin and either a small indistinct nucleolus or no nucleolus. The cytoplasm is moderate in amount and lightly basophilic, often with poorly defined margins. Anisokaryosis and anisocytosis are mild.

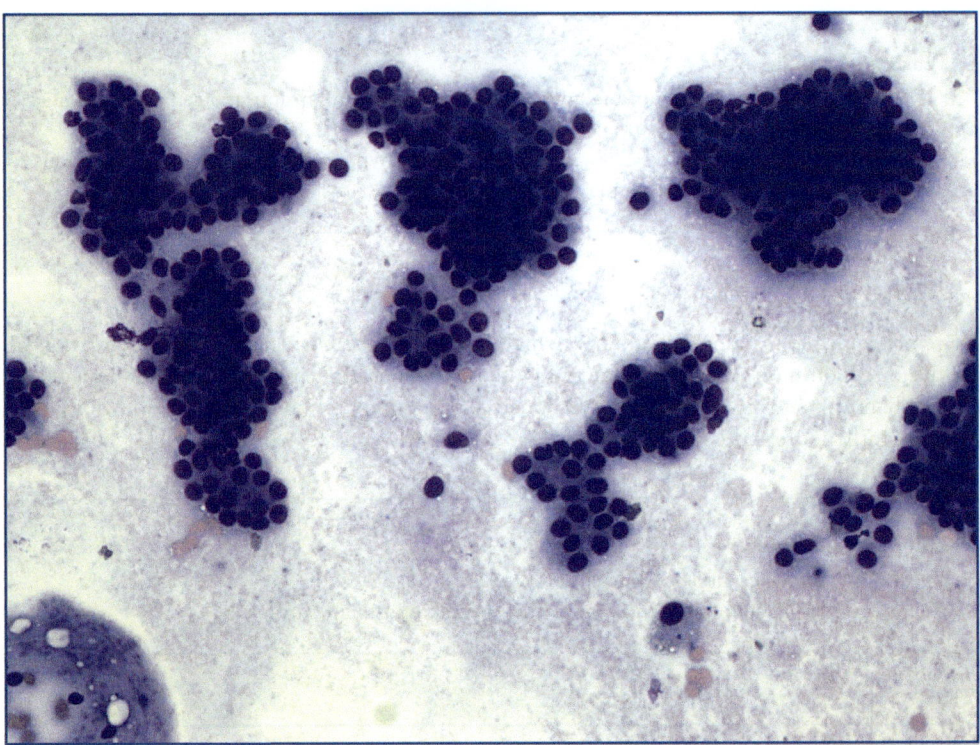

**Fig. 8.30.** Dog. Anal sac adenocarcinoma. Neoplastic cells are arranged in cohesive clusters. Wright-Giemsa.

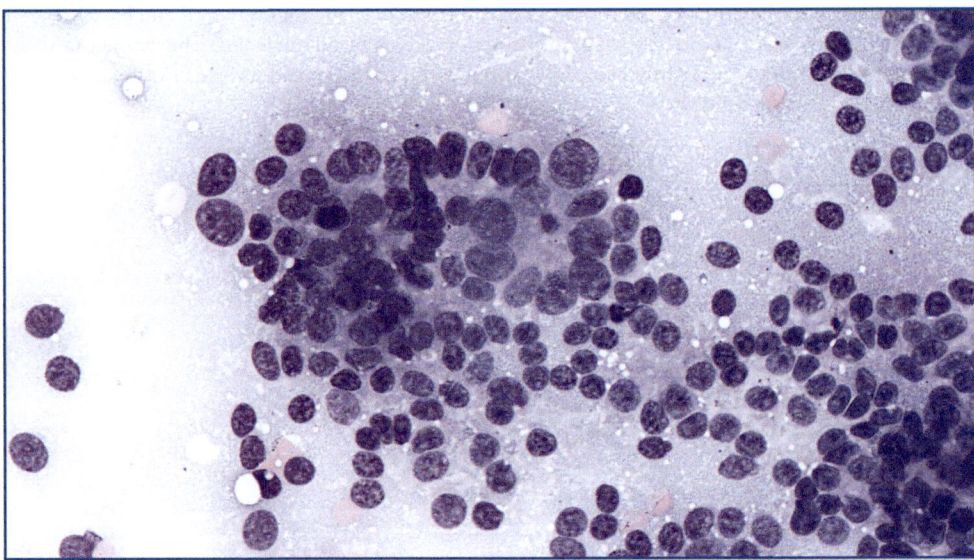

**Fig. 8.31.** Dog. Anal sac adenocarcinoma. Note a rosette-like/acinoid arrangement in the centre of the photograph. Wright-Giemsa.

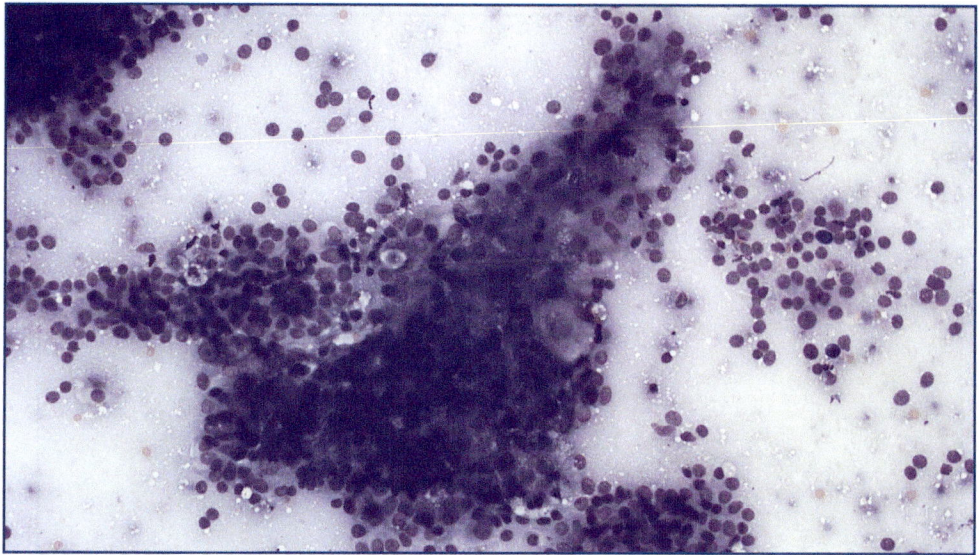

**Fig. 8.32.** Dog. Anal sac adenocarcinoma. Predominance of cuboidal epithelial cells with a high N:C ratio and poorly defined cell margins. Note the presence of large apocrine epithelial cells with a more abundant amount of cytoplasm. Occasionally, these cells may resemble perianal gland epithelial cells, though they do not have the typical fine grainy texture of the cytoplasm. Wright-Giemsa.

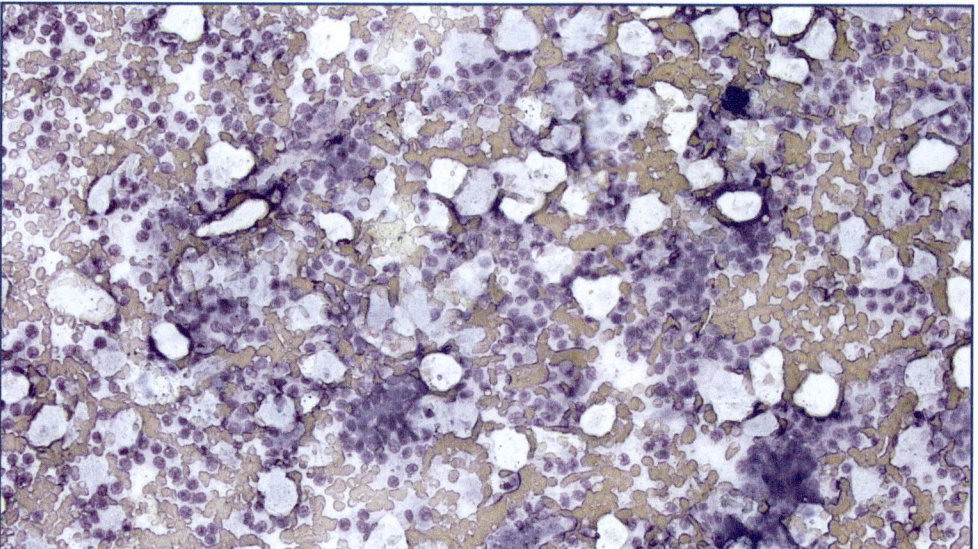

**Fig. 8.33.** Dog. Anal sac adenocarcinoma and impacted anal sac. Note the neoplastic apocrine epithelial cells admixed with numerous anucleated squamous epithelial cells. Wright-Giemsa.

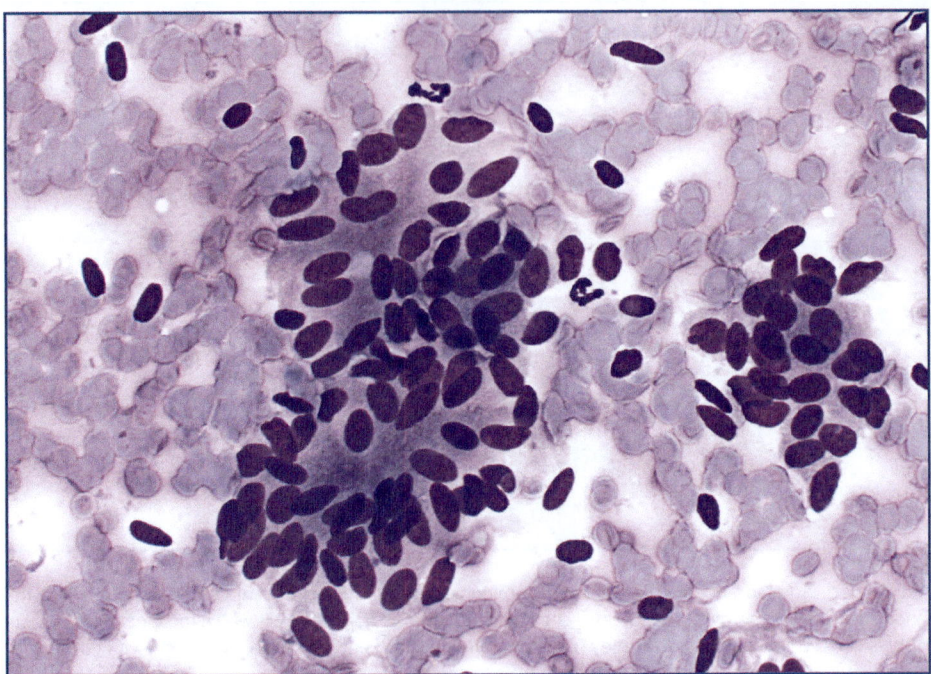

**Fig. 8.34.** Dog. Anal sac adenocarcinoma, spindle cells (atypical) variant. Neoplastic epithelial cells are in a cohesive cluster but have an elongated, spindloid shape. Wright-Giemsa. (*Courtesy of Hiroki Sakai, Gifu University, Japan.*)

## Further reading

Pradel, J., Berlato, D., Dobromylskyj, M. and Rasotto, R. (2018) Prognostic significance of histopathology in canine anal sac gland adenocarcinomas: preliminary results in a retrospective study of 39 cases. *Veterinary and Comparative Oncology* 16(4), 518–528.

Sakai, H., Murakami, M., Mishima, H., Hoshino, Y., Mori, T., Maruo, K. and Yanai, T. (2012) Cytologically atypical anal sac adenocarcinoma in a dog. *Veterinary Clinical Pathology*, 41(2), 291–294.

Shoied, A.M. and Hanshaw, D.M. (2009) Anal sac gland carcinoma in 64 cats in the United Kingdom (1995–2007). *Veterinary Pathology* 46, 677–683.

## 8.6   Clear Cell Adnexal Carcinoma (Dog)

Adnexal tumour without definitive apocrine, sebaceous or follicular differentiation. It arises in the dermis and can extend into the subcutaneous adipose tissue.

### Clinical features
- Rare tumour described only in dogs.
- Due to the paucity of reported cases in literature, there is no information on age, sex or breed predisposition and anatomical site predilection.
- Most of the cases described in the literature are slow growing.
- Local recurrence after surgery occurs rarely and metastasis to the draining lymph nodes is uncommon.

## Cytological features
- Cellularity is variable.
- Background: this is one of the most characteristic cytological features of this tumour. It contains a large amount of lacy, grey to amphophilic to basophilic, amorphous material representing the cytoplasmic content of the ruptured neoplastic cells. It can be variably haemodiluted.
- Cells exfoliate individually, in cohesive clusters or loose aggregates.
- Cells are often large. Morphology can vary from polygonal to oval and spindle shaped.
- Nuclei are round, occasionally oval, central and have coarse chromatin. They often contain one to multiple prominent nucleoli.
- The cytoplasm is variable in amount, often abundant with poorly defined margins. It is lightly grey-basophilic and may contain eosinophilic stippling, occasionally forming small needle-shaped pink structures. Cytoplasmic rarefaction can be observed.
- Rarely, the neoplastic cells contain melanin granules.
- Anisokaryosis and anisocytosis are often prominent. Multinucleated cells can be found (up to 10–15 nuclei).
- Necrosis and calcification might be observed.

### Differential diagnoses
- Poorly differentiated sebaceous carcinoma
- Sarcoma (including liposarcoma)
- Balloon cell melanoma

### Pearls and Pitfalls
- The name of this tumour derives from the fact that, on histopathology, the cells typically have a 'clear' and vacuolated cytoplasm.
- The misclassification of this tumour in favour of an erroneous diagnosis of sarcoma or melanoma can lead to inappropriate case management, as sarcomas and melanomas have a higher metastatic tendency and may have a worse prognosis.
- In some cases, immunohistochemistry is required for a definitive diagnosis.

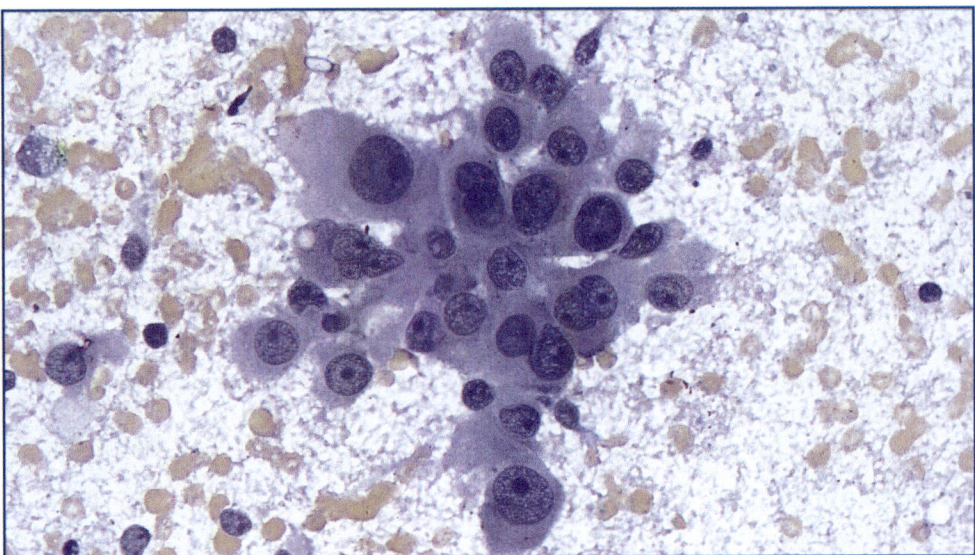

**Fig. 8.35.** Dog. Clear cell adnexal carcinoma. Note the typical lacy, grey to amphophilic to basophilic, amorphous material present in the background. Cells are polygonal to spindloid and arranged in a cohesive cluster. Anisokaryosis and anisocytosis are prominent and binucleation is observed. Wright-Giemsa.

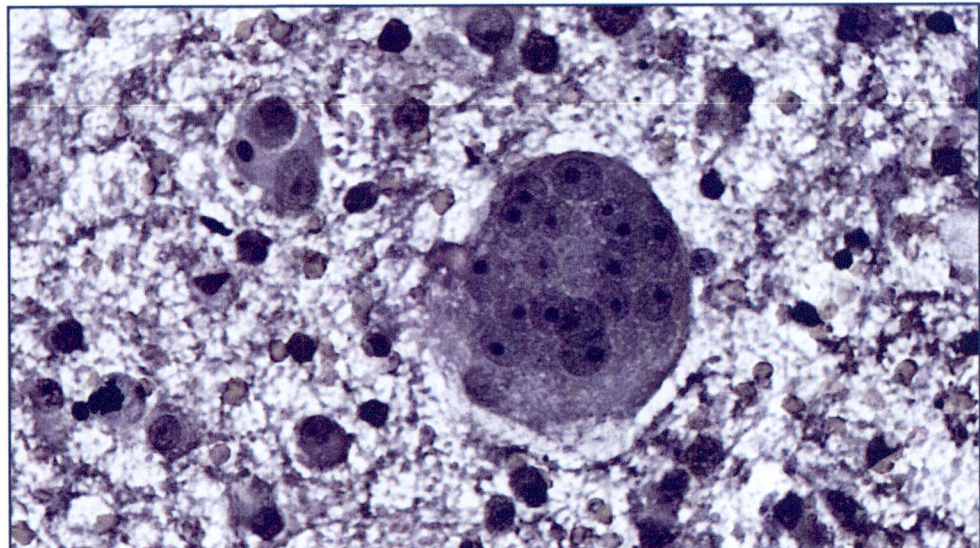

**Fig. 8.36.** Dog. Clear cell adnexal carcinoma. Large multinucleated cells can be observed in this tumour. Wright-Giemsa.

## Further reading

Piviani, M., Sánchez, M.D. and Patel, R.T. (2012) Cytologic features of clear cell adnexal carcinoma in 3 dogs. *Veterinary Clinical Pathology* 41(3), 405–411.

## 8.7   Merkel Cell Tumour

Neuroendocrine tumour originating from mechanoreceptors present in the epidermis and follicular epithelium. Also known as Merkel cell carcinoma.

### Clinical features

- Very rare neoplasm observed in middle-aged or older dogs and cats.
- Lesions usually appear as single, variable sized, firm, intradermal, flesh-coloured red nodules or plaques. The overlying skin may be alopecic and ulcerated. In cats, head and neck seem to be preferred locations.
- Usually benign in dogs. In cats, the clinical outcome may vary among cases. Tumours with high mitotic activity are often associated with a poorer prognosis, due to strong tendency towards local recurrence and regional lymph node and pulmonary metastases.

### Cytological features

- Cellularity is variable, often high.
- Background: pale basophilic and proteinaceous and variably haemodiluted.
- Neoplastic cells may appear as bare nuclei. When intact, they are round, cuboidal to polygonal and often in cohesive clusters.
- Nuclei are round to oval, central to eccentric with granular chromatin. Nucleoli are round and variably visible.
- The cytoplasm is scant, lightly to moderately basophilic, with variably defined borders.
- Cytological features of atypia are mild to moderate; binucleated cells and mitotic figures may be seen.

**Differential diagnoses**
- Metastatic neuroendocrine tumour
- Thyroid adenoma/carcinoma
- Cutaneous lymphoma (large cell type)

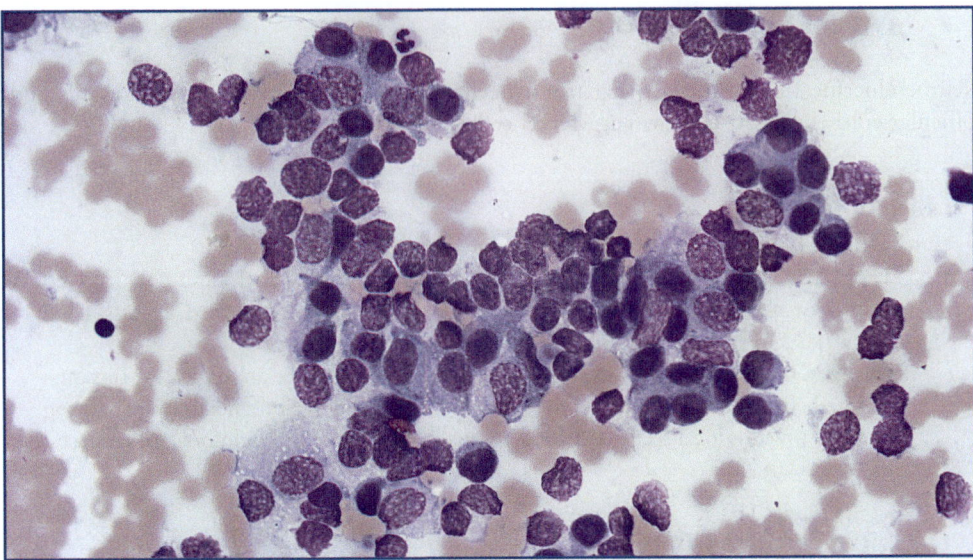

**Fig. 8.37.** Dog. Merkel cell tumour. Cells are relatively uniform in size and shape and have a high N:C ratio. Cell borders are poorly defined. Nuclei are round, with a finely stippled to granular chromatin and inconspicuous nucleoli. The cytoplasm is scant and pale basophilic. Wright-Giemsa.

## Further reading

Dohata, A., Chambers, J.K., Uchida, K., Nakazono, S., Kinoshita, Y., Nibe, K. and Nakayama, H. (2015) Clinical and pathologic study of feline Merkel cell carcinoma with immunohistochemical characterisation of normal and neoplastic Merkel cells. *Veterinary Pathology* 47(6), 1090–1094.

Sumi, A., Chambers, J.K., Doi, M., Kudo, T., Omachi, T. and Uchida K. (2018) Clinical features and outcomes of Merkel cell carcinoma in 20 cats. *Veterinary Comparative Oncology* 16(4), 554–561.

## 8.8 Diagnostic Algorithms

As discussed at the beginning of this chapter, on cytology some cutaneous epithelial tumours can share similar cellular and morphological features. Lesions that may show overlapping cytological findings include follicular cysts and tumours, sweat gland tumours and basal cell tumours. The following algorithms may help to refine the final diagnosis.

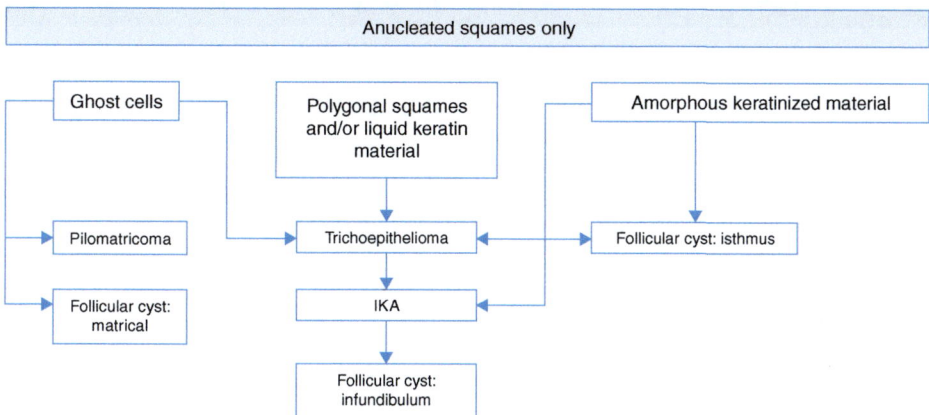

**Fig. 8.38.** Diagnostic algorithm to be used if only anucleated squamous epithelial cells exfoliate upon aspiration.

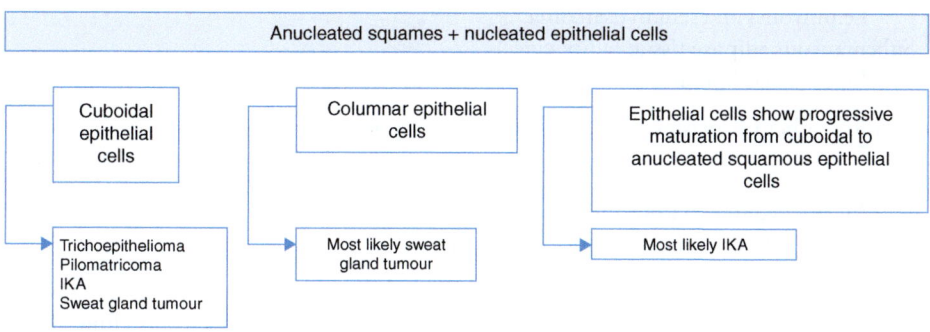

**Fig. 8.39.** Diagnostic algorithm to be used when both anucleated squamous epithelial cells and nucleated epithelial cells are present.

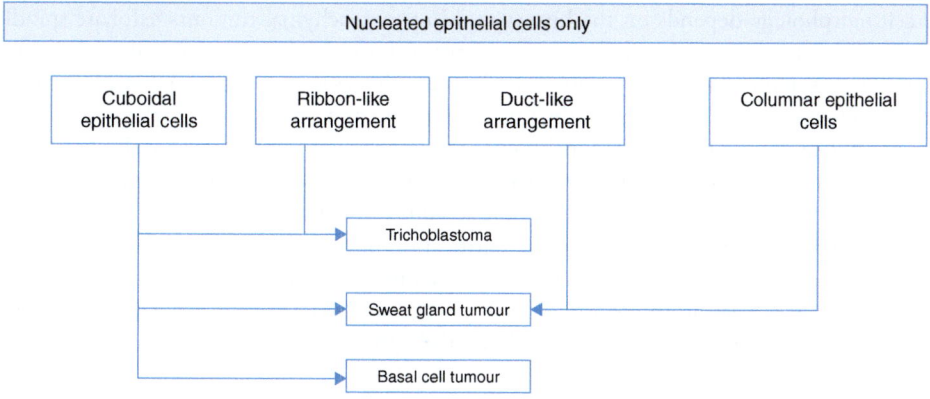

**Fig. 8.40.** Diagnostic algorithm to be used when only nucleated epithelial cells are present.

# Mesenchymal Tumours and Other Neoplasms

Mesenchymal tumours originate in the dermis and in the subcutaneous tissue. They can be classified based on the cell type they arise from:

- Connective tissue (fibrocytes/fibroblasts):
    - Fibroma and fibrosarcoma.
    - Myxoma and myxosarcoma.
    - Keloidal fibroma and fibrosarcoma.
- Vessels (endothelial cells and perivascular cells):
    - Haemangioma and haemangiosarcoma.
    - Perivascular wall tumours (PWTs).
- Nerves:
    - Peripheral nerve sheath tumours (PNSTs) including schwannoma.
- Smooth muscle cells of vessels and hair follicles:
    - Leiomyoma and leiomyosarcoma.
- Subcutaneous adipose tissue (adipocytes):
    - Lipoma and liposarcoma.

By extension, other neoplasms included in this category are:

- Melanocytes:
    - Melanocytoma and melanoma.
- Langerhans cells and interstitial dendritic cells:
    - Histiocytic disorders.

In this chapter, rhabdomyoma and rhabdomyosarcoma are discussed briefly, as clinically they may appear as subcutaneous masses, even if they arise from the beneath muscle layer.

## Cytological diagnosis of cutaneous mesenchymal lesions

The cell morphology depends on the histotype. Most mesenchymal tumours exfoliate spindle-shaped cells with oval nuclei and elongated cytoplasm forming characteristic tails; for this reason, the term spindle cell tumour is often used. In certain cases, specific cytological features are present, allowing the identification of the lineage of origin and a more detailed diagnosis. This is particularly true for neoplasms such as lipoma, liposarcoma and perivascular wall tumours. In other cases, cytological features are not considered typical for a specific mesenchymal neoplasm and a more generic term of soft tissue sarcoma or simply sarcoma is used.

It should also be emphasized that the identification of mesenchymal neoplasms is not free from interpretative doubts. Well-differentiated sarcomas may, in some instances, lack cytological criteria of atypia; on the contrary, in reactive fibroplasia and scar tissue, aspiration may exfoliate dysplastic fibroblasts, which could be misdiagnosed as neoplastic. In these cases, the clinical history and presentation (e.g. history of previous trauma/surgery, radiotherapy or evidence of a discrete mass) might help. The presence of a concurrent significant inflammation may also point in the direction of a reactive process; however, histopathology is often required for a definitive diagnosis.

## Soft tissue sarcomas (STSs)

This term refers to a specific group of mesenchymal tumours that arise from the soft tissues and that share a similar clinical behavior. STSs are locally infiltrative but have a low to moderate metastatic rate. The group of STSs includes:

- Fibrosarcoma.
- Myxosarcoma.
- Peripheral nerve sheath tumours.
- Perivascular wall tumours.
- Liposarcoma.
- Anaplastic sarcoma with giant cells/undifferentiated pleomorphic sarcoma.

Other sarcomas originating from soft tissues, such as histiocytic sarcoma and haemangiosarcoma, are conventionally excluded from this category because of their distinctive morphological features and more aggressive clinical behaviour.

## Grading of soft tissue sarcomas

The histopathological grading system for canine soft tissue sarcomas has a clinical significance and is able to predict local recurrence and development of metastasis. It is based on degree of cell differentiation, mitotic count and evidence of necrosis. These aspects can also be identified on cytology; however, a validated cytological grading system is not available at the present time.

# 9.1 Mesenchymal Tumours

## Fibroma and fibrosarcoma

Tumours originating from fibrocytes and fibroblasts of dermis and subcutis.

### Clinical features

- Fibroma:
    - Uncommon in dogs, accounting for less than 2% of all skin tumours. It is rare in cats.
    - It occurs in middle-aged or older animals.
    - It may present at any site but legs, head and trunk are preferred locations.
    - Masses are generally single, small, round to oval, intradermal or subcutaneous.
    - Fibroma is slow-growing and complete surgical excision is considered curative.
    - Over-represented canine breeds: Rhodesian Ridgeback, Dobermann, Boxer.
- Fibrosarcoma:
    - Uncommon in dogs; relatively frequent in cats, in which it represents up to 17% of all skin and subcutaneous tumours.
    - Fibrosarcoma belongs to the category of soft tissue sarcomas.
    - In cats, fibrosarcoma is often observed as a variant of the injection-site sarcoma.
    - Age: mostly seen in adult dogs and cats (average age of 9 years); however, it may also occur in very young animals.
    - Preferred locations include head, legs and trunk. In cats, it commonly occurs in the interscapular area (injection-site fibrosarcoma) and ear pinnae.
    - Masses are often large, well circumscribed or infiltrating. They may be multilobulated, often cystic and ulcerated.
    - Fibrosarcoma has a tendency to be infiltrative and recurrent especially in high-grade forms, but metastases are uncommon.
    - Over-represented canine breeds: mostly large-breed dogs, including Golden Retriever, Dobermann, Brittany, Gordon Setter, Irish Wolfhound.
    - No predisposed feline breeds reported.

## Cytological features

- Fibroma:
    - Cellularity is very low and aspirates might not be diagnostic.
    - Background: clear and variably haemodiluted.
    - Cells usually exfoliate individually or in very loose aggregates.
    - Cells are small, spindle shaped and fusiform and generally uniform.
    - Nuclei are oval, with finely stippled to lacy chromatin.
    - The cytoplasm forms one or two slender and pale basophilic tails with poorly demarcated margins.
- Fibrosarcoma:
    - Cellularity is variable, often high.
    - Background: variably haemodiluted.
    - Aspirates are composed of mesenchymal cells, which exfoliate individually or in aggregates. Storiform patterns may be observed. Neoplastic cells may be embedded in pink amorphous material.

- Cells are spindle shaped to plump-oval.
- Nuclei are generally large, round to oval and with coarse to granular chromatin. Nucleoli are often prominent.
- The cytoplasm is lightly to moderately basophilic and has poorly defined margins. It can contain clear vacuoles and/or pink granules.
- Cytological features of atypia can be marked and include anisokaryosis, anisocytosis, multiple prominent nucleoli (e.g. round, oval, angular or irregular), anisonucleoliosis, multinucleation and atypical mitotic figures.

---

**Differential diagnoses**
- Fibroma:
  - Collageneous hamartoma
  - Reactive fibroplasia/scar tissue formation
  - Keloidal fibroma (rare)
- Fibrosarcoma:
  - Reactive fibroplasia/scar tissue formation
  - Soft tissue sarcoma of other origin
  - Nodular fasciitis (rare)
  - Keloidal fibrosarcoma (rare)

---

**Pearls and Pitfalls**
- Fibrosarcoma lacks specific morphological features and can mimic other sarcomas. For this reason, a generic diagnosis of (soft tissue) sarcoma is often made on cytology. A definitive confirmation of fibrosarcoma relies on histopathology.
- An uncommon variant called *canine maxillary well-differentiated sarcoma* has been described in Golden Retrievers and other large-breed dogs. Despite being an extremely well-differentiated neoplasm with minimal nuclear pleomorphism, this neoplasm is often rapidly growing and progressive infiltrative. It presents with a swelling of the maxillary or mandibular region.
- A rare hereditary syndrome of multiple fibromas in the dermis and subcutis has been reported in German Shepherd Dogs. Clinical presentation is characterized by numerous small dermal nodules, especially on limbs, ears and back. It is important to recognize this syndrome, as it has often been associated with multiple renal cysts, adenomas or adenocarcinomas and uterine leiomyomas.

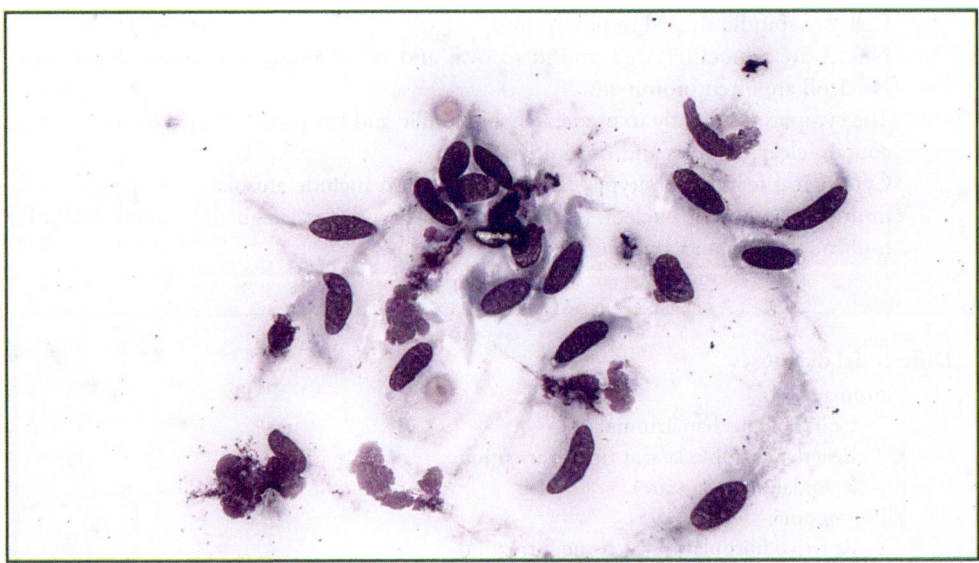

**Fig. 9.1.** Dog. Fibroma. Wright-Giemsa.

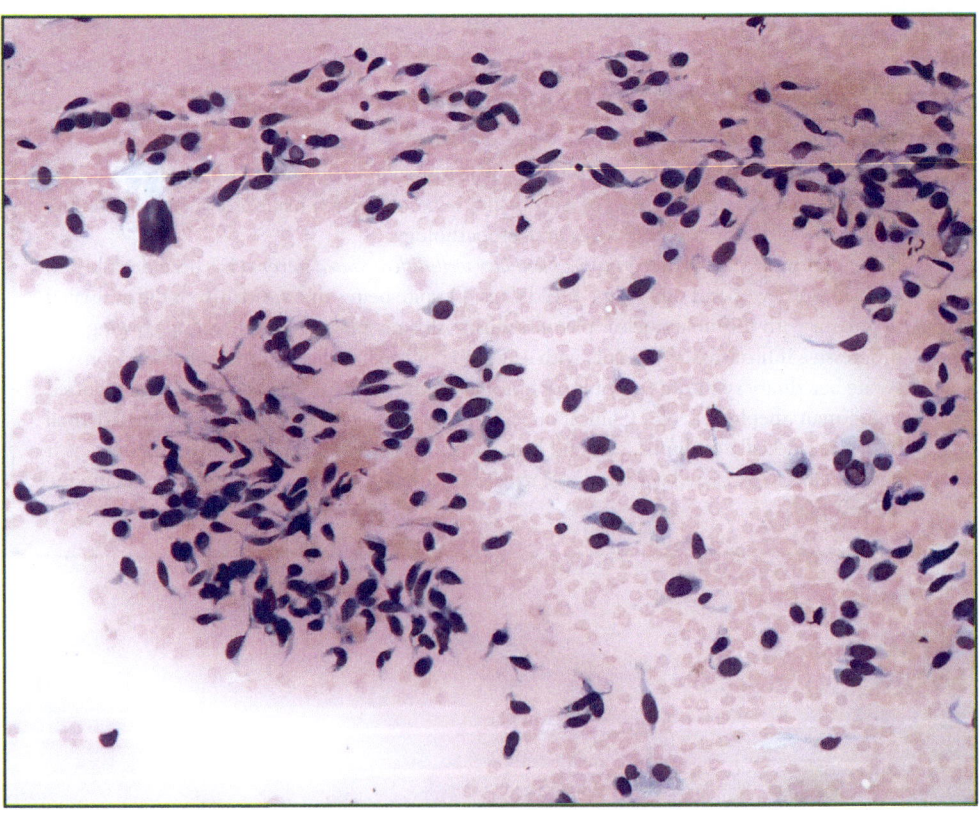

**Fig. 9.2.** Dog. Fibrosarcoma. Individualized, well-differentiated and slender spindle cells. Wright-Giemsa.

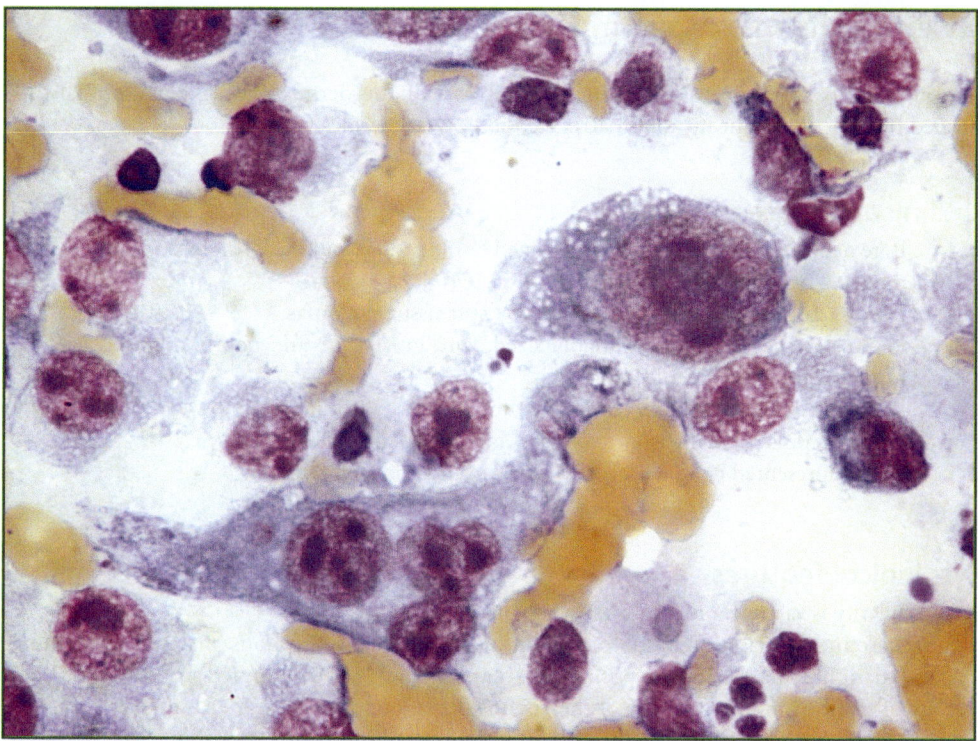

**Fig. 9.3.** Dog. Fibrosarcoma. Mesenchymal cells show marked cytological features of atypia including marked anisokaryosis, prominent nucleoli and multinucleation. Wright-Giemsa.

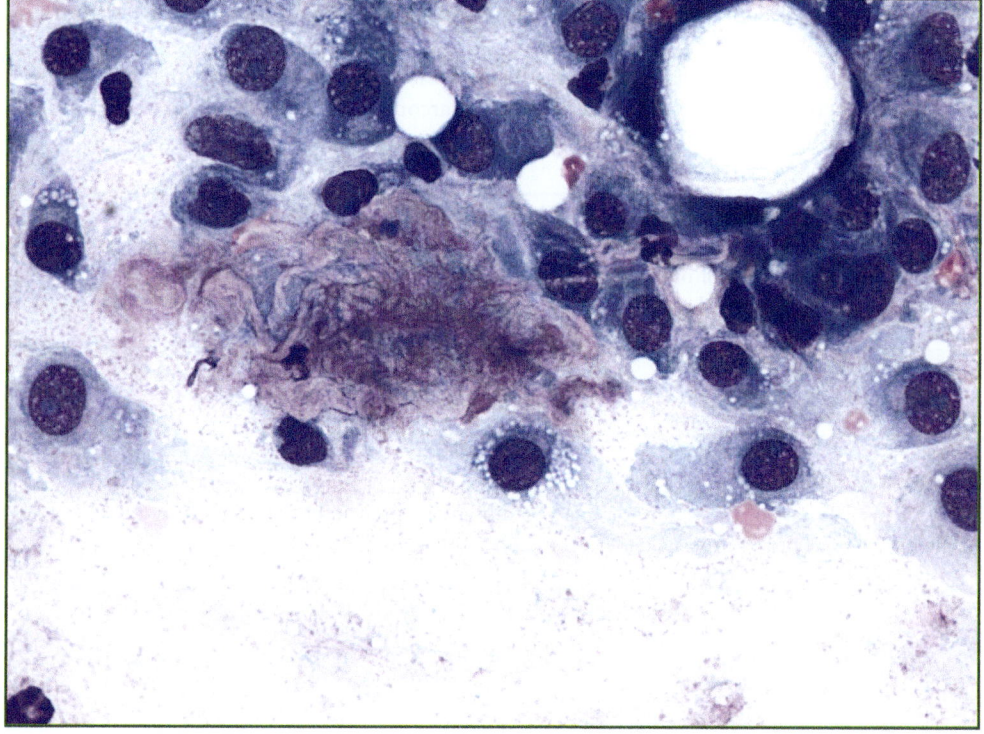

**Fig. 9.4.** Dog. Fibrosarcoma. Mesenchymal cells show moderate cytological features of atypia and are admixed with eosinophilic amorphous material (matrix). Wright-Giemsa.

# Myxoma and myxosarcoma

Tumours originating from fibrocytes and fibroblasts of the dermis and subcutis and distinguished by their abundant myxoid matrix rich in polysaccharides (mucin).

## Clinical features
- Rare neoplasms observed in middle-aged or older dogs and cats. They account for less than 1% of all skin tumours.
- Myxosarcoma belongs to the category of soft tissue sarcomas.
- Lesions are usually single, variably sized, soft, grey-white and poorly defined. They may exude a clear mucoid fluid.
- It is most commonly observed in the subcutis of the trunk and limbs.
- Myxosarcoma is locally infiltrative and metastases are rare.
- Over-represented canine breeds: Basset Hound and Dobermann.

## Cytological features
- Cellularity is variable, often low, especially in benign forms.
- Background: variable amount of viscous, eosinophilic amorphous material containing abundant mucin (Alcian blue positive). It may be variably haemodiluted and red blood cells are often lined in rows because of the viscous background.
- Neoplastic cells are fusiform to stellate and loosely arranged in aggregates. They are often embedded in abundant pink matrix.
- Nuclei are oval and the chromatin is granular to coarse. Prominent nucleoli may be seen in myxosarcoma.
- The cytoplasm is lightly basophilic, often forming one or two tails projecting away from the nucleus.
- Cytological features of atypia, multinucleation and mitoses are often observed in myxosarcoma.
- The distinction between myxoma and myxosarcoma can be difficult on the basis of cytology alone.

**Differential diagnoses**
- Soft tissue sarcoma of other origin
- Liposarcoma (myxoid variant)

**Pearls and Pitfalls**

Cytological smears of these tumours may be difficult to prepare because the slimy texture of the sample may prevent the specimen from adhering to the slide.

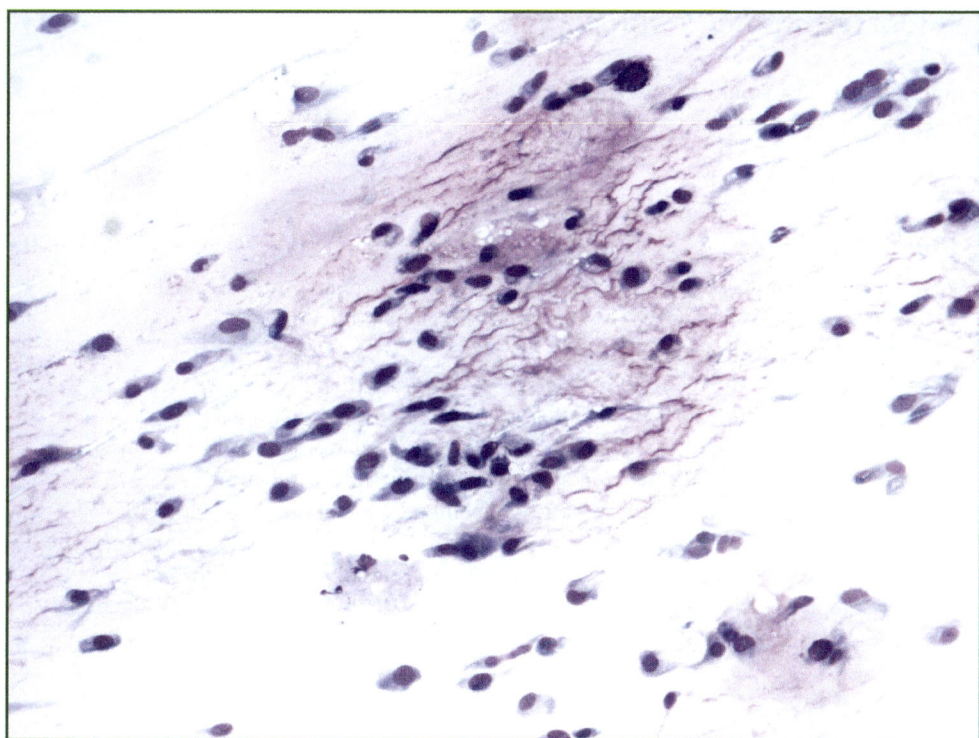

**Fig. 9.5.** Dog. Myxoma. Uniform elongated spindle cells admixed with mucinous material. Wright-Giemsa.

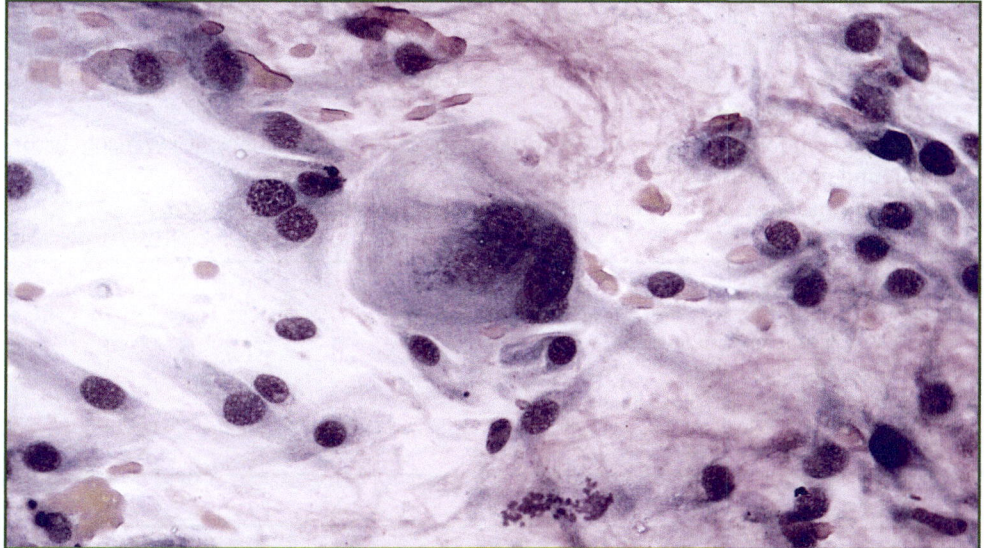

**Fig. 9.6.** Dog. Myxosarcoma. Plump and elongated mesenchymal cells admixed with abundant myxoid matrix. Multinucleation and a mitosis are seen. Wright-Giemsa.

# Keloidal fibroma and fibrosarcoma

Tumours of mesenchymal origin characterized by deposition of a large amount of hyalinized collagen.

## Clinical features

- Very uncommon skin neoplasms in dogs. Not reported in cats, except for a single case of vaccine-associated fibrosarcoma with keloidal differentiation.
- Male dogs appear over-represented.
- Masses may develop at any site.
- They can be spontaneous or secondary to trauma or inflammation.
- Most tumours present as single, rarely multiple, nodular or plaque-like lesions. They are often poorly demarcated and arise in the dermis and/or subcutis.
- The vast majority of keloidal tumours are benign (keloidal fibroma). However, keloidal fibroma may undergo malignant transformation into keloidal fibrosarcoma. The differentiation between these two forms is based on histological findings.
- Over-represented canine breeds: shorthaired dogs, including Rhodesian Ridgeback.

## Cytological features

- Cellularity is variable, from low to high.
- Background: clear and variably haemodiluted.
- Presence of numerous elongated fragments of pink, glassy bundles of collagen fibrils.
- Aspirates yield variable numbers of mesenchymal cells that are slender, spindle shaped, often arranged in large aggregates and embedded in collagenous material.
- Nuclei are oval, with finely stippled to lacy chromatin. Nuclear features of atypia may be observed in malignant forms.
- The cytoplasm forms one or two tails with poorly demarcated margins. It is variably basophilic and occasionally contains pink granules.
- Mast cells, macrophages/histiocytes and eosinophils may be occasionally seen.

### Differential diagnoses

- Mast cell tumour with numerous collagen fibrils
- Collagenous hamartoma
- Reactive fibroplasia/scar tissue
- Soft tissue sarcoma of other origin

### Pearls and Pitfalls

Hyalinized collagen in keloidal fibroma/sarcoma is bright magenta, glassy, lacking of distinct linear fibrils, and is more striking than the amorphous, wispy, eosinophilic to magenta matrix frequently associated with other soft tissue sarcomas. In mast cell tumours, the collagen flame figures are less eosinophilic and more fibrillar.

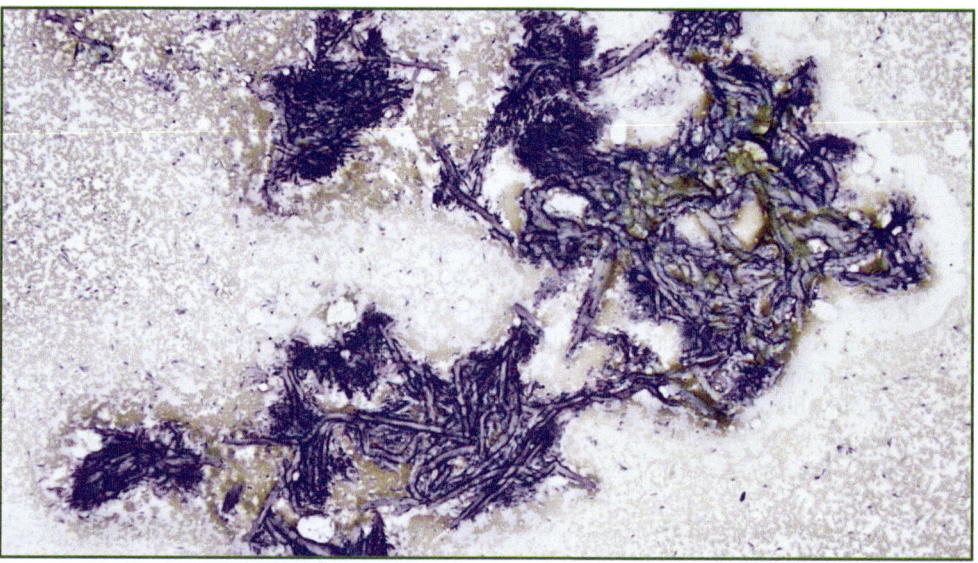

**Fig. 9.7.** Dog. Keloidal fibrosarcoma. Large amounts of hyalinized collagen fibrils associated with slender neoplastic spindle cells. Wright-Giemsa.

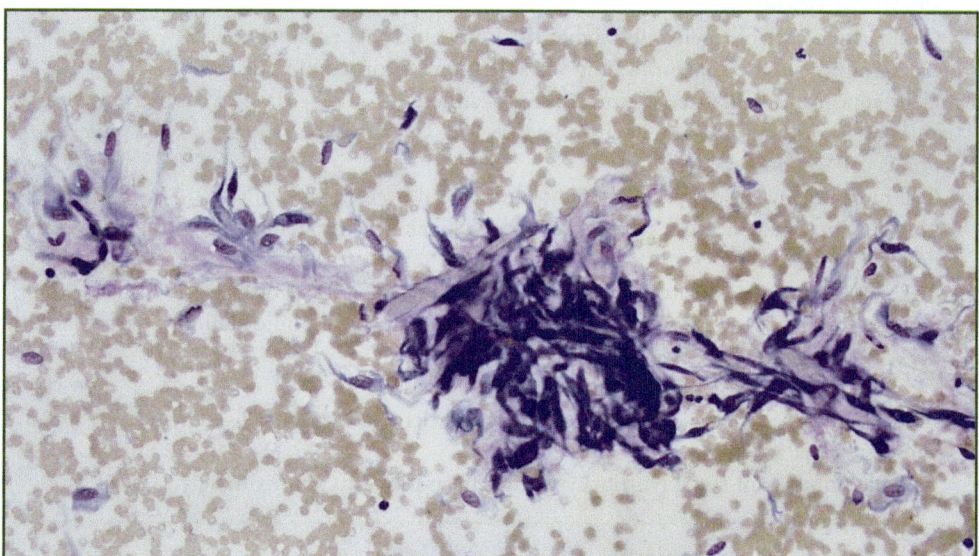

**Fig. 9.8.** Dog. Keloidal fibrosarcoma. Mesenchymal cells are uniform and do not show significant features of atypia. Wright-Giemsa.

## Further reading

Gumber, S. and Wakamatsu, N. (2011) Vaccine-associated fibrosarcoma with keloidal differentiation in a cat. *Journal of Veterinary Diagnostic Investigations* 23(5), 1061–1064.

Little, L.K. and Goldschmidt, M. (2007) Cytologic appearance of a keloidal fibrosarcoma in a dog. *Veterinary Clinical Pathology* 36(4), 364–367.

Mikaelian, I. and Gross, T.L. (2002) Keloidal fibromas and fibrosarcomas in the dog. *Veterinary Pathology* 39, 149–153.

# Perivascular wall tumours (PWTs)

Group of tumours that arise from cells of the perivascular wall and adventitia.

## Clinical features
- Relatively common mesenchymal neoplasms affecting dogs, in particular large breeds, middle-aged to older subjects. Very rare in cats.
- They belong to the class of soft tissue sarcomas.
- Recent studies have shown that PWTs represent a spectrum of tumours arising from various cells of the perivascular wall and adventitia, such as pericytes and myopericytes. These tumours include haemagiopericytoma, myopericytoma, myoma, angioleiomyoma, angiomyofibroblastoma, angiofibroma and glomus tumours.
- They often appear as solitary lesions, with predilection for limbs and joints. Gross appearance is variable, often rubbery; macroscopically it may be confused for lipoma.
- PWTs are locally infiltrative with a relatively low metastatic risk.
- Good prognosis if associated with early diagnosis, small tumour size (< 5 cm), cutaneous/subcutaneous localization with no deeper involvement and clean surgical margins.

## Cytological features
- Cellularity is variable, generally higher than most mesenchymal tumours.
- Background: clear, often containing variable numbers of red blood cells.
- Cells appear individualized or form bundles adherent to the surface of capillaries. Perivascular or whorling arrangements can be observed. Cells may be associated with pink amorphous collagenous stroma.
- Cell morphology varies between wispy, plump-oval, stellate and veiled.
- Nuclei are generally medium sized and round, with granular chromatin and occasionally visible nucleoli.
- The cytoplasm is moderate in amount, moderately basophilic, often containing distinct, clear, round intracytoplasmic vacuoles and rarely small eosinophilic granules. Cells margins are often fringed.
- Cytological features of atypia are variable.
- Binucleated (insect-head cells) and multinucleated elements (crown cells) may be seen and are considered characteristic.
- Variable numbers of small lymphocytes have been found in approximately 10% of cases.

### Differential diagnoses
- Peripheral nerve sheath tumours (PNSTs), including schwannoma
- Soft tissue sarcoma of other origin
- Round cell tumour (including plasma cell tumour and cutaneous histiocytoma)

### Pearls and Pitfalls
Crown cells in PWTs are so called because they are characterized by having the nuclei arranged in a circle at the periphery of the cytoplasm, resembling a crown or wreath.

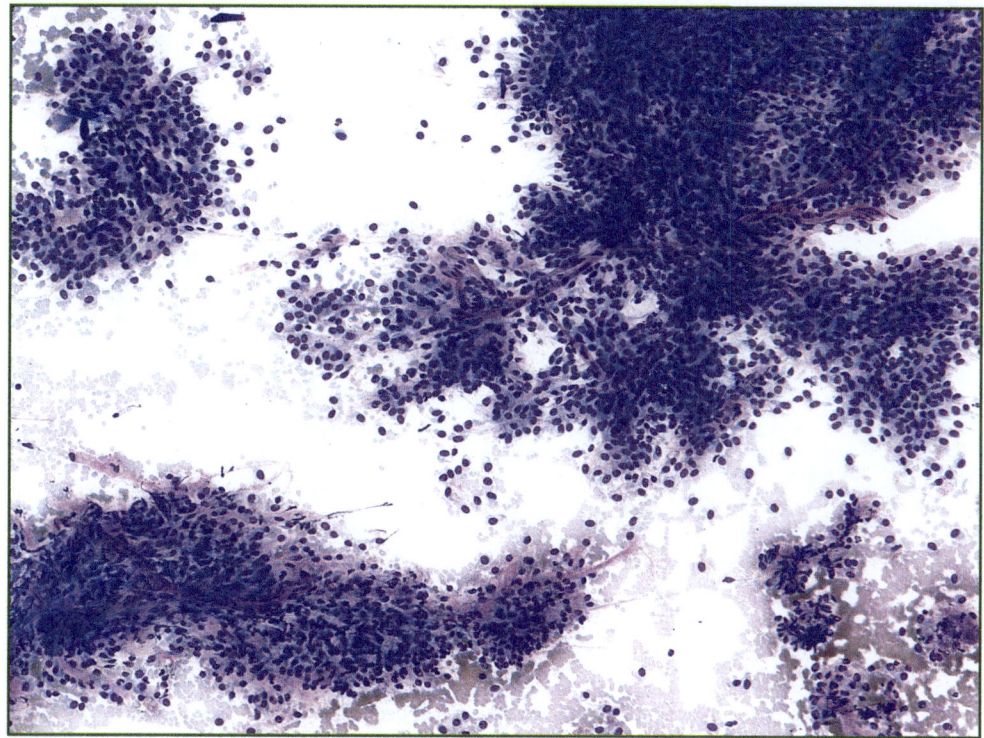

**Fig. 9.9.** Dog. Perivascular wall tumour. Neoplastic cells are arranged along linear streaming capillaries. Wright-Giemsa.

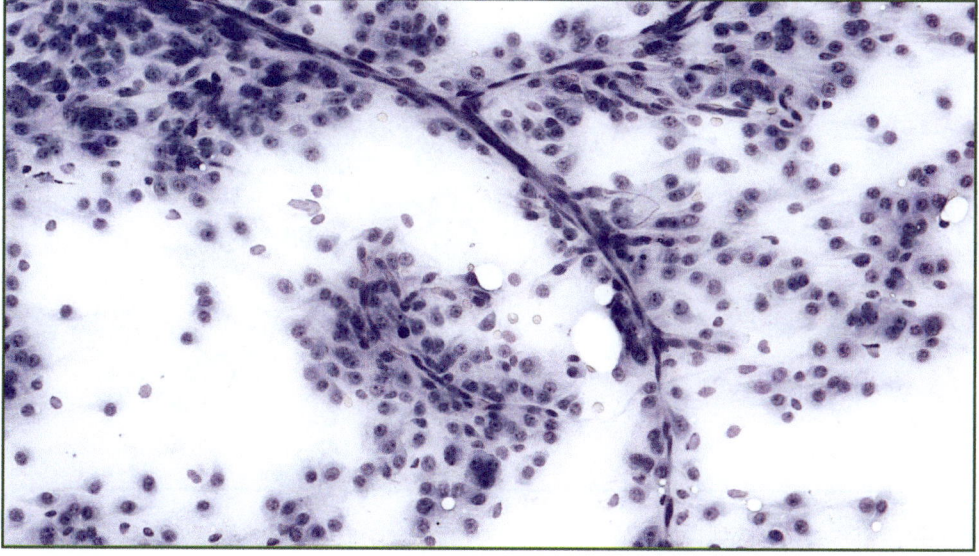

**Fig. 9.10.** Dog. Perivascular wall tumour. Neoplastic cells are arranged along linear streaming capillaries. Wright-Giemsa.

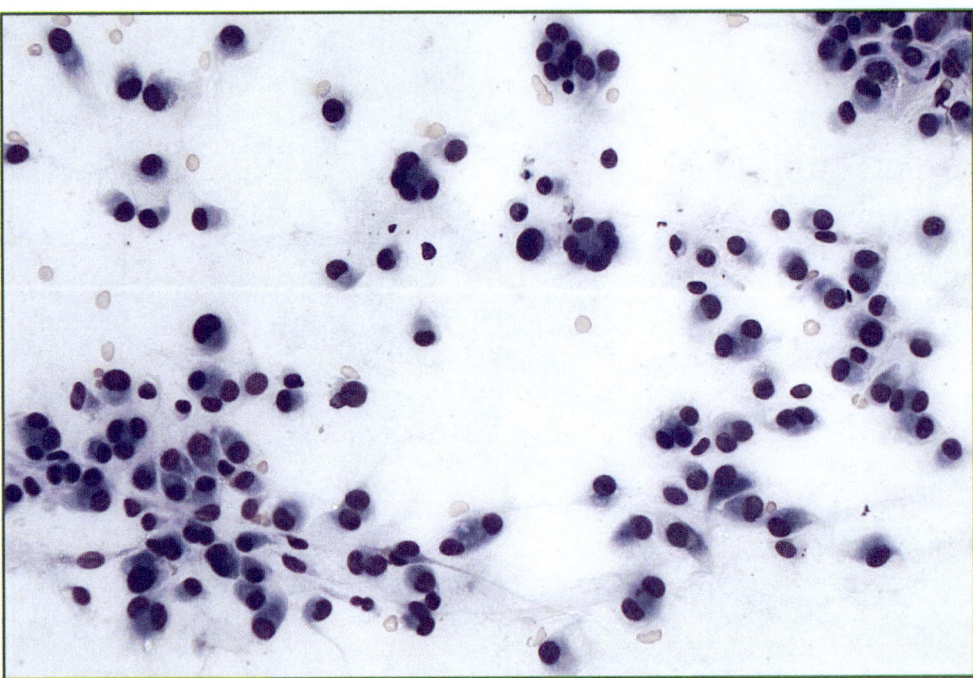

**Fig. 9.11.** Dog. Perivascular wall tumour. Neoplastic cells often appear binucleated and multinucleated (crown cells). Wright-Giemsa.

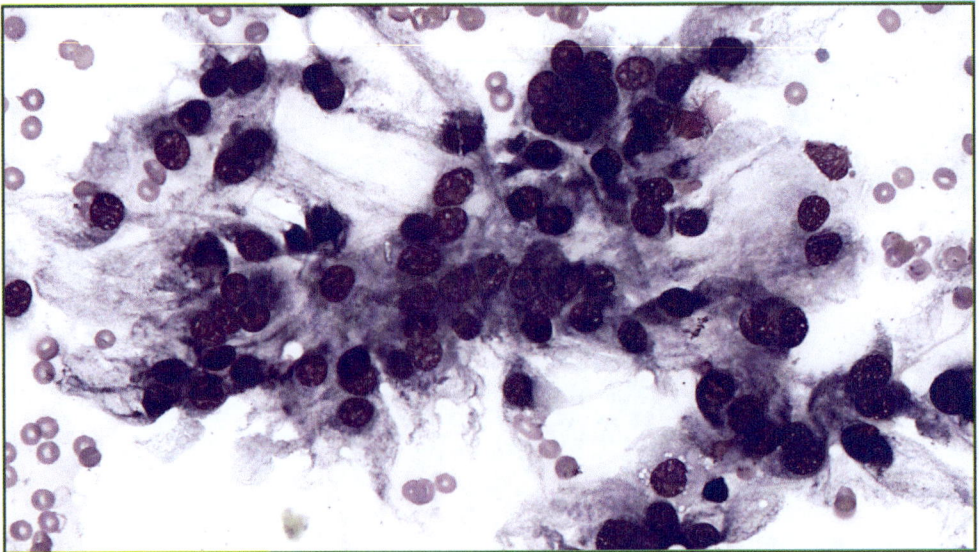

**Fig. 9.12.** Dog. Perivascular wall tumour. Note the perivascular whorling of neoplastic cells. Wright-Giemsa.

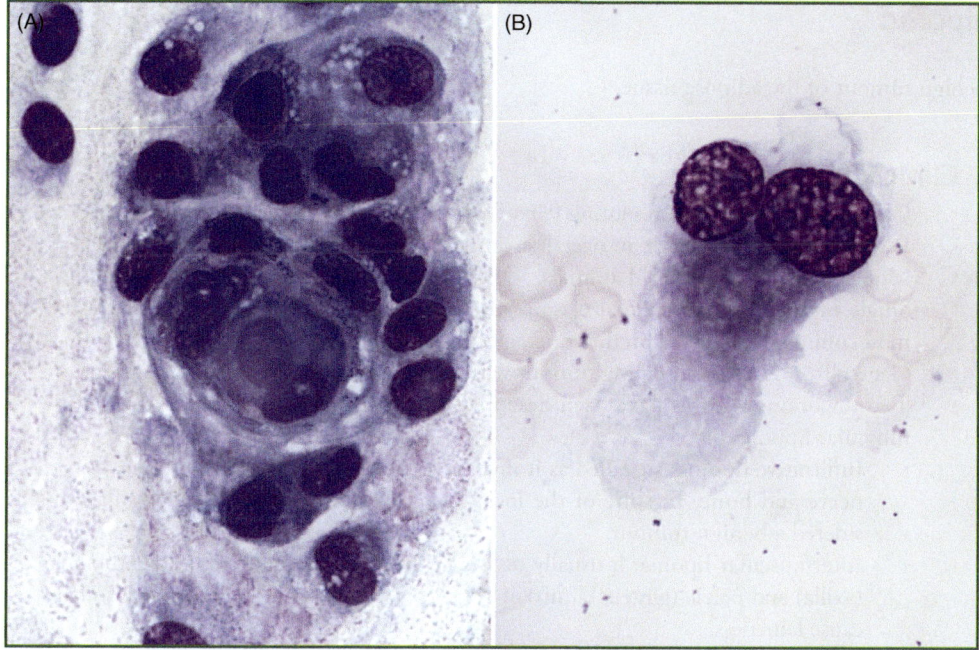

**Fig. 9.13.** Dog. Perivascular wall tumour. (A) Cell whirling. (B) Binucleated cell (insect face cell).

## Further reading

Avallone, G., Helmbold, P., Caniatti, M., Stefanello, D., Nayac, R.C. and Roccabianca, P. (2007) The spectrum of canine cutaneous perivascular wall tumours: morphologic, phenotypic and clinical characterisation. *Veterinary Pathology* 44(5), 607–620.

Avallone, G., Boracchi, P., Stefanello, D., Ferrari, R., Rebughini, A. and Roccabianca, P. (2014) Canine perivascular wall tumours: high prognostic impact of site, depth, and completeness of margins. *Veterinary Pathology* 51(4), 713–720.

Caniatti, M., Ghisleni, G., Ceruti, R., Roccabianca, P. and Scanziani, E. (2001) Cytological features of canine hae-mangiopericytoma in fine needle aspiration biopsy. *Veterinary Record* 149(8), 242–244.

Stefanello, D., Avallone, G., Ferrari, R., Roccabianca, P. and Boracchi, P. (2011) Canine cutaneous perivascular wall tumours at first presentation: clinical behaviour and prognostic factors in 55 cases. *Journal of Veterinary Internal Medicine* 25, 1398–1405.

# Lipoma

Benign tumour of the adipose tissue.

## Clinical features

- Common neoplasm, representing 9% of all skin and subcutaneous tumours in dogs. Less common in cats with an overall estimated incidence of 3–5%.
- More common in adult/old animals.
- Single or multiple, variable size, soft, often freely moveable, subcutaneous masses, most commonly observed on the trunk, gluteal region and proximal limbs.
- Generally, it is a slow-growing tumour with good prognosis after surgical excision.
- Two uncommon forms have been described in dogs and cats: infiltrative and inter-muscular lipomas.
  - Infiltrative lipoma: so called as it invades adjacent tissues such as muscle, fascia, nerve and bone. In spite of the local aggressive growth pattern, it is still considered a benign tumour.
  - Intermuscular lipoma: it usually occurs in the intermuscular area of the thoracic (axilla) and pelvic (gluteus) limbs of dogs. It is slow growing and can occasionally cause lameness.
  - Both infiltrative and intermuscular lipomas are cytologically similar to conventional lipomas and subcutaneous adipose tissue.
  - Their differentiation is based on clinical presentation, imaging and histopathology.

## Cytological features

- Cellularity is generally low.
- Background: clear, often containing variably sized clear lipid vacuoles and variably haemodiluted.
- Adipocytes can be seen individually or in aggregates.
- Cells are large, containing a single clear lipid vacuole occupying most of the cytoplasm.
- The nucleus is small, round to oval, hyperchromic and peripherally placed.
- Supporting stromal cells, collagen, capillaries and/or cartilage may be seen occasionally. When these components are abundant, the terms fibrolipoma, angiolipoma, angiofibrolipoma and chondrolipoma can be used.

## Variants

A new histological variant of lipoma has recently been described:

- Spindle cell lipoma:
  - Rare in dogs, not reported in cats.
  - It resembles an undifferentiated soft tissue sarcoma; differentiation is based on histopathological, histochemical and immunohistochemical findings.
  - Vacuolated spindle-shaped and plump cells are seen and are admixed with collagen, myxoid matrix and low numbers of mature adipocytes.

**Differential diagnosis**

Subcutaneous adipose tissue (accidental aspiration)

**Pearls and Pitfalls**

Aspirates from lipoma often contain variable amounts of lipid material. Slides often do not dry and have an oily appearance. The lipid component may dissolve during fixation in methanol-based fixatives and may detach the adipocytes from the slide, leaving an acellular smear. This can be prevented by: (i) heat fixation (unstained slide passed through a flame for a few seconds); (ii) using poly-L-lysine slides.

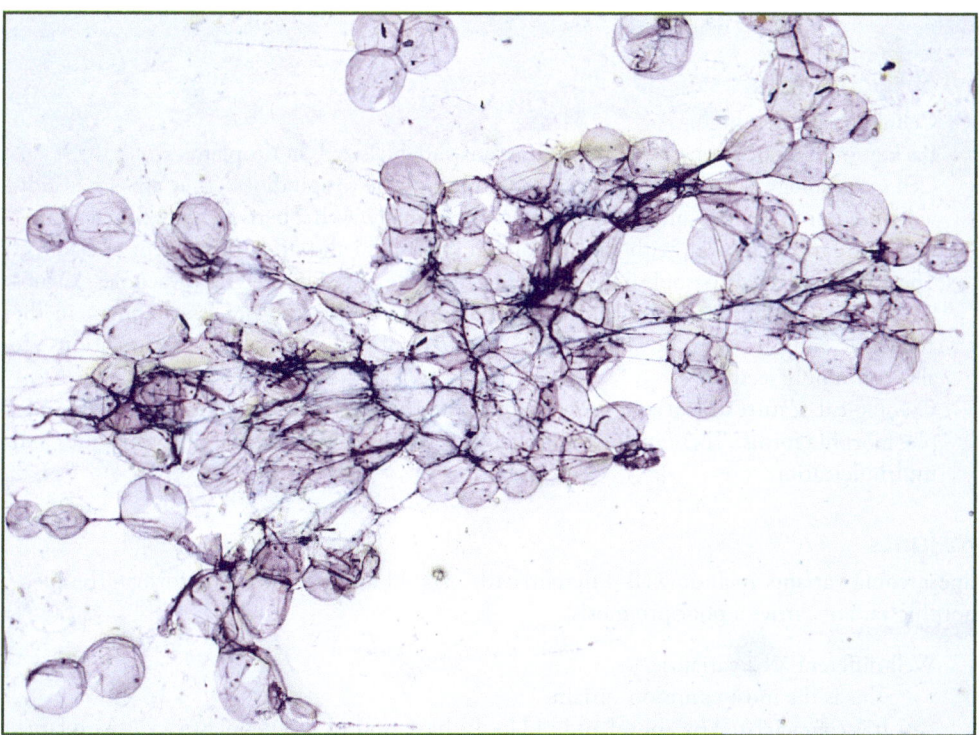

**Fig. 9.14.** Dog. Perivascular wall tumour. (A) Cell whirling. (B) Binucleated cell (insect face cell).

# Further reading

Avallone, G., Pellegrino, V., Muscatello, L.V., Sarli, G. and Roccabianca, P. (2017) Spindle cell lipoma in dogs. *Veterinary Pathology* 54, 792–794.

Case, J.B., MacPhail, C.M. and Whitrow, S.J. (2012) Anatomic distribution and clinical findings of intermuscular lipomas in 17 dogs (2005–2010). *Journal of American Animal Hospital Association* 48(4), 245–249.

Liggett, A.D., Frazier, K.S. and Styer, E.L. (2002) Angiolipomatous tumors in dogs and a cat. *Veterinary Pathology* 39, 286–289.

# Liposarcoma

Malignant tumour of the adipose tissue.

## Clinical features

- Rare tumour observed in older dogs and cats.
- In some cases, an association with glass foreign bodies and implanted microchips has been described in dogs.
- It belongs to the class of soft tissue sarcomas.
- Masses are usually solitary and firm. They occur more frequently on ventrum and extremities. Another relatively common primary location is the tongue.
- Locally invasive neoplasm with a low metastatic potential.
- Over-represented canine breeds: Shetland Sheepdog and Beagle.

## Cytological features

- Cellularity is often high.
- Background: clear, often containing numerous variably sized fat droplets.
- Cell morphology is variable. Cells vary from plump-oval to spindloid. They are either individualized or in poorly cohesive aggregates, occasionally with a perivascular arrangement.
- Nuclei are round to oval, with coarse granular chromatin and often prominent nucleoli.
- The cytoplasm is pale basophilic and contains multiple, variably sized lipid vacuoles. Vacuoles are more numerous in well-differentiated forms, whilst they are less frequent in the anaplastic and pleomorphic variants. Fine pink/eosinophilic cytoplasmic granulations are also commonly seen.
- Cytological features of atypia are variable, often marked, especially in anaplastic and pleomorphic forms. These include anisokaryosis, anisocytosis, atypical mitotic figures and multinucleation.

## Variants

Liposarcoma variants include well-differentiated, myxoid and pleomorphic forms. The pleomorphic variant carries a poor prognosis.

- Well-differentiated variant:
  - This is the most common variant.
  - It is characterized by abundant lipid in the background and neoplastic cells with large, clear lipid displacing and flattening the nucleus to the periphery.
- Myxoid variant:
  - Rare variant.
  - Neoplastic cells vary in shape. They are loosely embedded in a myxoid eosinophilic stroma that stains positive to Alcian blue.
- Pleomorphic variant:
  - Rare variant.
  - Cells are characterized by marked cellular atypia and bizarre binucleated or multinucleated cells.

**Differential diagnoses**

- Panniculitis/steatitis and fat necrosis
- Sarcoma of other origin
- Amelanotic and ballooning melanoma
- Granular cell tumour
- Sebaceous carcinoma
- Clear cell carcinoma
- Myxoma/myxosarcoma (for myxoid liposarcoma)
- Histiocytic sarcoma (for pleomorphic liposarcoma)

**Pearls and Pitfalls**

Sudan and Oil Red O stain can be used on unfixed slides to confirm the lipid origin of the intracytoplasmic vacuoles of neoplastic cells.

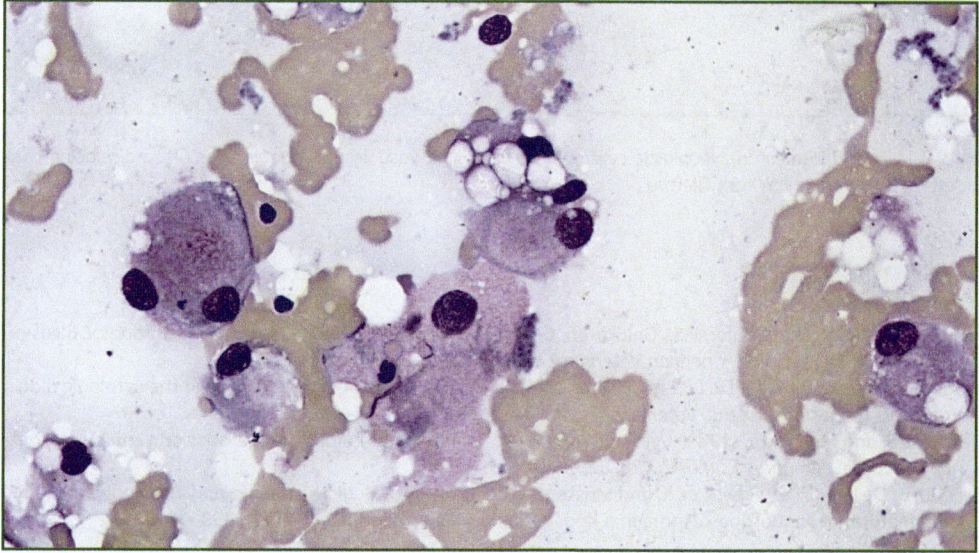

**Fig. 9.15.** Dog. Liposarcoma. Note the fine pink/eosinophilic cytoplasmic granulations within the neoplastic cells. Wright-Giemsa.

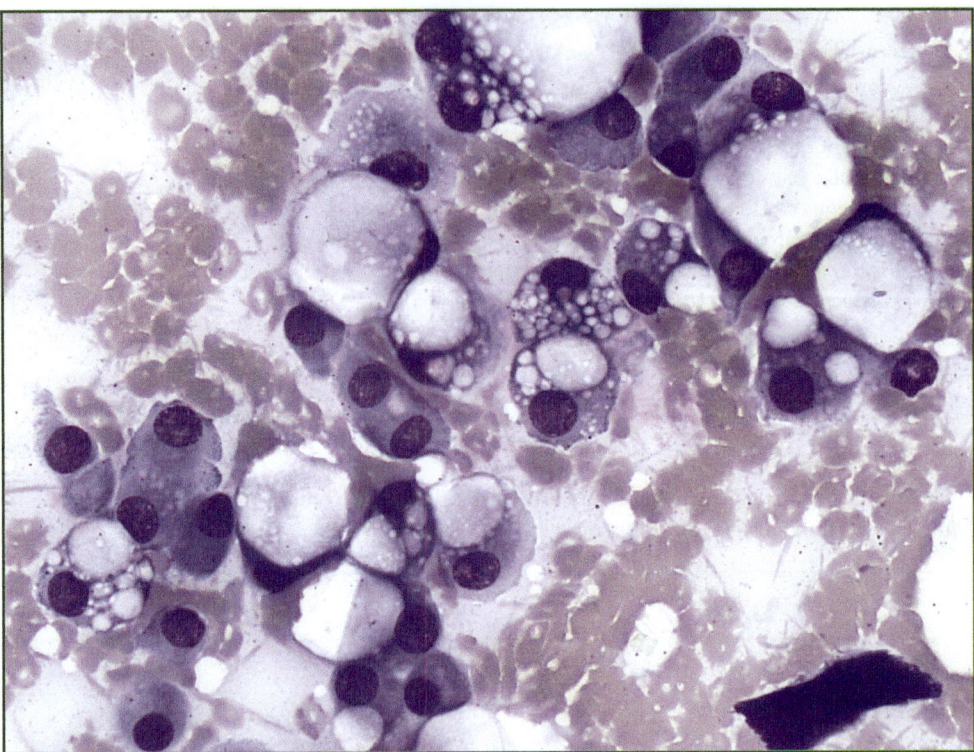

**Fig. 9.16.** Dog. Liposarcoma. Neoplastic cells contain clear lipid vacuoles of variable sizes often displacing the nucleus to the periphery. Wright-Giemsa.

## Further reading

Baez, J.L., Hendrick, M.J., Shofer, F.S., Goldkamp, C. and Sorenmo K.U. (2004) Liposarcomas in dogs: 56 cases (1989–2000). *Journal of American Veterinary Medical Association* 224(6), 887–891.

Masserdotti, C., Bonfanti, U., De Lorenzi, D. and Ottolini, N. (2006) Use of Oil Red O stain in the cytologic diagnosis of canine liposarcoma. *Veterinary Clinical Pathology* 35(1), 37–41.

Messick, J.B. and Radin, M.J. (1989) Cytologic, histologic, and ultrastructural characteristics of a canine myxoid liposarcoma. *Veterinary Pathology* 26, 520–522.

Piseddu, E., De Lorenzi, D., Freeman, K. and Masserdotti, C. (2011) Cytologic, histologic, and immunohistochemical features of lingual liposarcoma in a dog. *Veterinary Clinical Pathology* 40(3), 393–397.

# Haemangioma

Benign tumour arising from the vascular endothelium.

## Clinical features

- Common neoplasm in dogs, accounting for 4.5% of all skin neoplasms; rare in cats, with an estimated incidence of 1.5–2%.
- Cutaneous haemangioma is mostly observed in adult/old patients. Similar lesions have also been described in young animals, but may represent vascular malformations rather than a true neoplasm.
- Well-demarcated dermal or subcutaneous mass, often bright red to dark brown. It may be cavitated, contain variable amounts of blood, and ulcerated.
- Haemangioma occurs at any anatomical site.
- Solar-induced form has been described in light-skinned, short-haired dog breeds and cats. This is more often localized in glabrous skin areas and may be multiple.
- Generally it is a slow-growing process.
- Over-represented canine breeds: Airedale Terrier, Gordon Setter, Boxer, Soft-coated Wheaten Terrier, Wire Fox Terrier, Golden Retriever, Old English Sheepdog, English Springer Spaniel, German Shepherd Dog, Whippet, Bloodhound, Saluki and Pointer.

## Cytological features

- Cellularity is generally low and fine-needle aspirate can be non-diagnostic.
- Background: heavily haemodiluted. Platelets are not commonly seen.
- Low numbers of endothelial cells and capillary structures might exfoliate. Endothelial cells are spindle shaped, occasionally plump, and have oval, often folded nuclei.
- Macrophages can be present, often showing erythrophagia or containing haemosiderin and/or haematoidin crystals, indicative of previous haemorrhage.

## Variants

Several variants of haemangioma have been described in the literature and include cavernous, infiltrative, capillary, arteriovenous, granulation tissue type, spindle-cell, epithelioid and solar-induced forms. Differentiation is based on histopathology.

**Differential diagnoses**
- Iatrogenic haemorrhage
- Haematoma
- Vascular malformation
- Well-differentiated haemangiosarcoma

**Pearls and Pitfalls**
Cytological diagnosis can be difficult because of the marked haemodilution of the sample and the relatively low numbers of neoplastic cells harvested. Histopathology is often needed for a definitive diagnosis.

# Haemangiosarcoma

Malignant tumour of vascular endothelium.

## Clinical features

- Accounts for slightly less than 1% of cutaneous and subcutaneous tumours in dogs and 2.8% in cats.
- Average age for cutaneous and subcutaneous haemangiosarcoma is 9–11 years in both dogs and cats.
- Single, well-demarcated dermal or subcutaneous mass, often bright red to dark brown, soft to firm; it may be cavitated, contain variable amounts of blood, and ulcerated. More aggressive forms may present with poorly defined borders and may infiltrate adjacent tissues.
- Cutaneous and subcutaneous haemangiosarcoma in dogs may be solitary or part of a multicentric syndrome involving internal organs (e.g. spleen, liver). In cats it may be seen on the abdominal region, head (eyelid, pinnae), distal limbs and paws.
- A solar-induced form has been observed in both dogs (short-haired, light-skinned breeds) and cats (white-haired males). It mostly occurs on glabrous skin areas.
- Cutaneous haemangiosarcomas are less aggressive than their visceral counterparts, with lower metastatic potential and longer survival time.
- Histological location may have a prognostic significance in dogs, with dermal haemangiosarcoma being associated with prolonged survival time when compared with forms that invade the subcutaneous tissues or muscles.
- Over-represented canine breeds: short-haired, light-skinned dog breeds (e.g. Greyhound, Whippet) and American Pit Bull Terrier.

## Cytological features

- Cellularity is variable, often low.
- Background: heavily haemodiluted with large numbers of red blood cells; platelets are not commonly seen.
- Aspirates are composed of variably but often large spindle-shaped mesenchymal cells. They occur singly or in small aggregates.
- Nuclei are round to oval, medium to large. The chromatin is clumped or coarse. Nucleoli may be multiple, prominent, round to irregularly shaped.
- The cytoplasm is moderate to abundant and variably basophilic. It is often elongated and can contain small punctate clear vacuoles.
- Cells can exhibit erythrophagia and/or contain blue-black granules of haemosiderin.
- Anisokaryosis, anisocytosis and degree of pleomorphism are variable, often marked.
- Mitotic figures, including atypical forms, can be found.
- Low numbers of inflammatory cells, including macrophages containing red blood cells/ haemosiderin/haematoidin crystals may be observed.
- Haematopoietic precursors may occasionally be found (less commonly than in visceral forms).

## Variants

Different variants of haemangiosarcoma have been described in the literature and include epithelioid, solar-induced and anaplastic forms. Differentiation is made on histopathology; however, some variants may be suspected on cytology, such as the epithelioid haemangiosarcoma.

- **Epithelioid variant**
  Neoplastic endothelial cells resemble epithelial cells (hence epithelioid) for appearance and arrangement. They occasionally contain intracytoplasmic clear vacuoles.

**Differential diagnosis**
Sarcoma of other origin

**Pearls and Pitfalls**
- Aspiration from cavitated areas of the mass can lead to excessive haemodilution of the sample and inadequate nucleated cellularity. Sampling from solid areas of the mass may increase the likelihood of harvesting neoplastic cells.
- Lymphangiosarcomas are neoplasms of the lymphatic vessels. They are uncommon and may appear cytologically similar to haemangiosarcomas. These tumours often arise in the subcutis of ventral midline and limbs and form poorly demarcated, sometimes oedematous masses. In cats, this form is also known as *feline ventral abdominal angiosarcoma*.

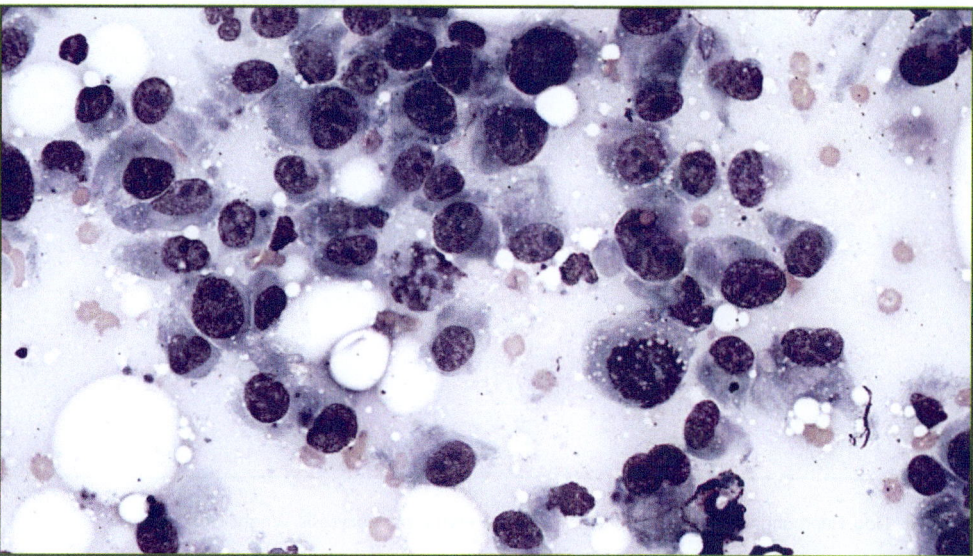

**Fig. 9.17.** Dog. Haemangiosarcoma. Neoplastic cells show marked anisokaryosis, prominent and multiple nucleoli and atypical mitoses. Wright-Giemsa.

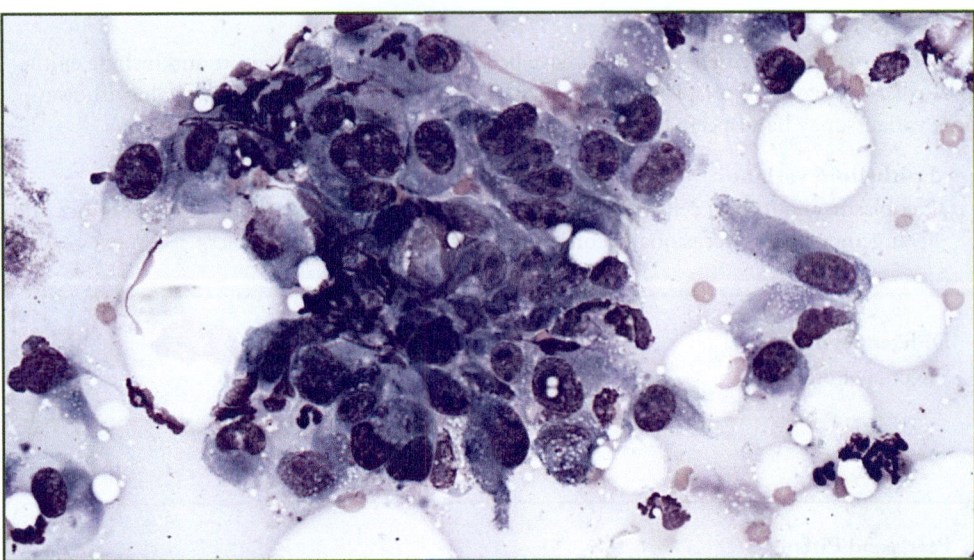

**Fig. 9.18.** Dog. Haemangiosarcoma. Neoplastic cells have an epithelioid appearance and are arranged in an apparently cohesive aggregate. Wright-Giemsa.

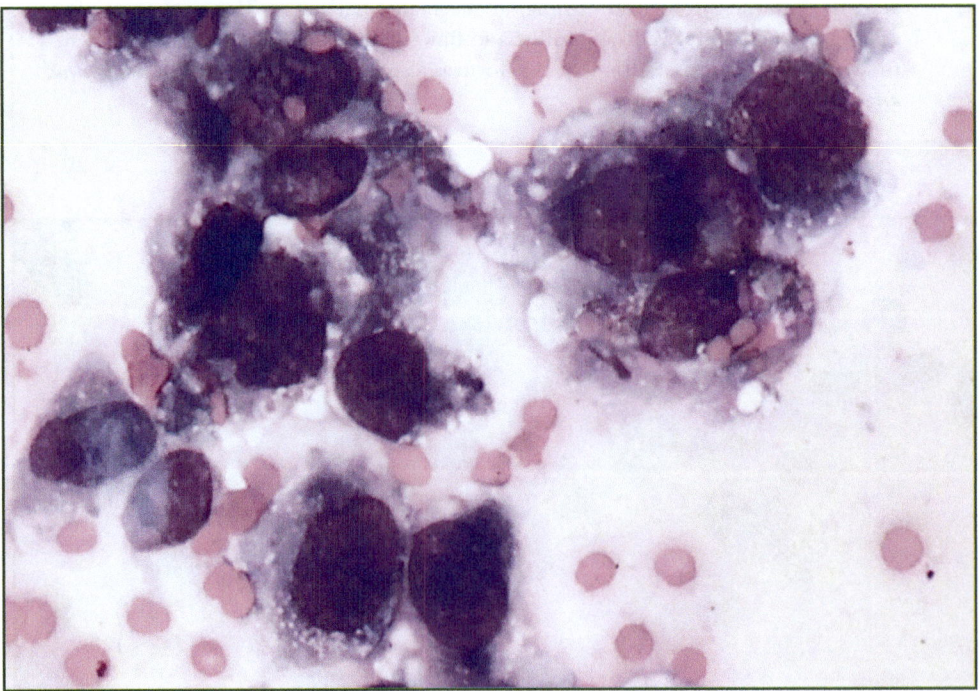

**Fig. 9.19.** Dog. Haemangiosarcoma. Neoplastic cells show erythrophagocytosis. Wright-Giemsa.

# Further reading

Ward, H., Fox, L., Calderwood, M.B., Hammer, A.S. and Couto, C.G. (1994) Cutaneous hemangiosarcoma in 25 dogs: a retrospective study. *Journal of Veterinary Internal Medicine* 8(5), 345–348.

Warren, A.L. and Summers, B.A. (2007) Epithelioid variant of hemangioma and hemangiosarcoma. *Veterinary Pathology* 44(1), 14–24.

# Anaplastic sarcoma with giant cells and pleomorphic sarcoma

Group of poorly differentiated sarcomas characterized by the presence of multinucleated giant cells. Also called undifferentiated pleomorphic sarcoma or malignant fibrous histiocytoma (MFH).

## Clinical features

- Uncommon tumour with a reported incidence of less than 0.5% and 0.9% of all cutaneous neoplasms in dogs and cats, respectively.
- Average age is 8 and 10 years in dogs and cats, respectively; however, lesions may be seen in young animals.
- Females are more frequently affected than males (2:1).
- In dogs, it may arise in the skin as a single expansive lesion, or it may be part of a multiorgan disease.
- In cats it is considered a variant of the vaccine-associated sarcoma but it may occur also in non-vaccine sites.
- Solitary or multiple, variably sized, unencapsulated, poorly defined, subcutaneous and dermal masses. In dogs, most tumour masses are located on extremities and periarticular regions (e.g. elbow and stifle); in cats, the few cases described are located on the extremities and abdomen, unless part of the injection site sarcoma complex.
- These tumours are locally infiltrative. Localized forms have a better prognosis if treated early with wide surgical excision. Prognosis of disseminated forms is poor. Behavioural differences may reflect the different cellular origin of these neoplasms.
- Over-represented canine breeds: Rottweiler, Golden Retriever and Flat-coated Retriever.

## Cytological features

- Cellularity is variable, often high.
- Background: clear to lightly basophilic and variably haemodiluted.
- Neoplastic cells are pleomorphic, often rounded to elongated and often exfoliate individually; they may occasionally form poorly cohesive groups with a storiform arrangement.
- Nuclei are round to oval, often large, with coarse, granular or clumped chromatin. Multiple prominent and irregularly shaped nucleoli are frequently seen.
- The cytoplasm is basophilic, moderate in amount and forms small cytoplasmic tails. It may contain clear intracytoplasmic vacuoles.
- Large to very large multinucleated cells (up to 30 nuclei) are frequently seen in the sarcoma with giant cells variant.
- Cytological features of atypia are often marked and include anisocytosis, anisokaryosis, variation in nucleus-to-cytoplasm ratio and often irregular mitotic figures.

## Variants

Two main histological variants have been reported in the skin/subcutis of domestic animals. The most relevant features of these variants can also be recognized on cytology.

- Storiform pleomorphic type:
  - This is the most common form in dogs.
  - Neoplastic cells are spindle shaped (fibroblast-like cells) and arranged in storiform patterns.
  - There are also histiocytoid cells, which often display karyomegaly and multinucleation.
  - Mixed inflammatory cells are often present.
- Giant cell type:
  - This is the most common variant in cats.
  - It exfoliates multinucleated giant cells admixed with mononuclear histiocytoid elements.
  - Inflammatory cells are not a consistent feature of this variant.

---

**Differential diagnoses**
- Histiocytic sarcoma
- Sarcoma of other origin

---

**Pearls and Pitfalls**
- Initially thought to be one neoplasm with different variants, recent studies have shown this likely represents an umbrella, descriptive and more general term that includes anaplastic versions of several mesenchymal and histiocytic tumours. This includes a tumour of myofibroblast origin that is analogous to the human malignant fibrous histiocytoma (MFH).
- When the tumour arises at the level of a joint, immunohistochemistry is required to differentiate it from other neoplasms typical of this location, including histiocytic sarcoma and synovial sarcoma.

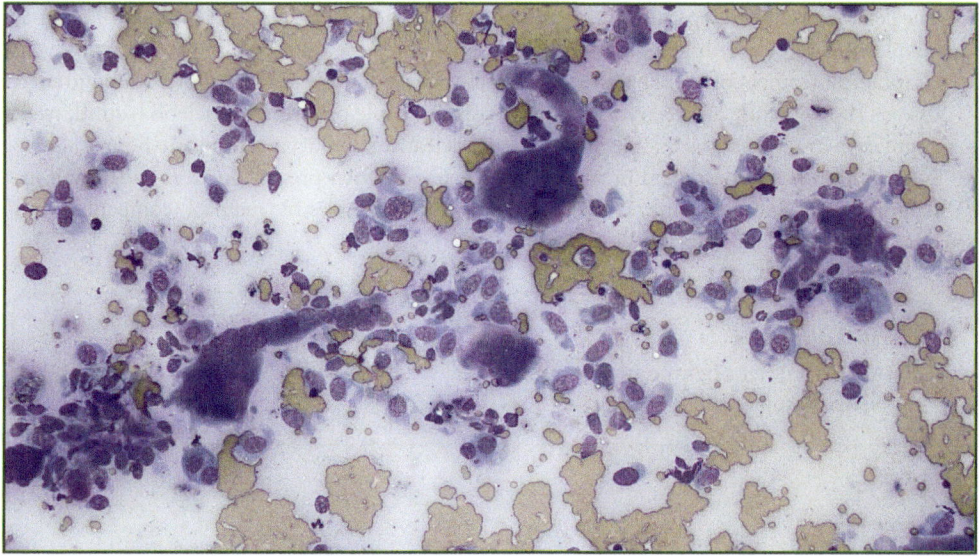

**Fig. 9.20.** Cat. Anaplastic sarcoma with giant cells. Wright-Giemsa.

# Injection site sarcoma

Malignant tumour of different lineage that may develop at sites of previous injections.

## Clinical features

- It occurs in a range from 1:1000 to 1:10,000 tumours per vaccinated cat. It is very rare in dogs.
- Age in cats: as young as 3 years of age with an average of 8–10 years.
- Described after the injection of vaccines, long-acting antibiotics, steroids, non-absorbable material and microchip implant. Chronic inflammatory stimulation can stimulate proliferation of fibroblasts and myofibroblasts and subsequent malignant transformation through multiple cytokines and growth factors.
- Injection-site sarcoma can have different histotype origins. The most common forms are fibrosarcoma, anaplastic sarcoma with giant cells, osteosarcoma, chondrosarcoma, rhabdomyosarcoma and undifferentiated sarcoma.
- It presents as variably sized, firm, poorly demarcated, often multilobulated, cutaneous or subcutaneous nodules at sites commonly used for injections, such as neck, interscapular space, thorax, lumbar region, flanks and limbs. Lesions often contain a cystic centre containing a watery or mucinous fluid.
- Local recurrence after surgery is common due to the infiltrative growth pattern. Metastatic risk is low to moderate and in cats ranges from 10% to 28%. Metastases tend to occur late in the course of the disease and primarily affect regional lymph nodes, mediastinum and lungs.

## Cytological features

- The cellularity is variable, from low to high.
- Background: clear to lightly basophilic and variably haemodiluted. Depending on the histotype of the tumour, variable amounts of matrix (e.g. osteoid, chondroid, collagen, etc.) can be present.
- The cell morphology depends on the histotype of the neoplastic cells (refer to fibrosarcoma, anaplastic sarcoma with giant cells, etc.).
- Cytological features of atypia are variable, often marked, especially in poorly differentiated forms. These include anisokaryosis, anisocytosis, multiple prominent nucleoli (round, oval, angular or irregular), anisonucleoliosis, multinucleation and atypical mitotic figures.
- Neutrophils, macrophages and/or small lymphocytes are often present due to a concurrent inflammation. Macrophages may contain grey/brown intracytoplasmic material (compatible with injected material). Necrosis can be observed.

### Differential diagnoses

- Sarcoma of other origin
- Reactive fibroplasia

**Pearls and Pitfalls**

- The cytological distinction between injection-site sarcoma and severe reactive fibroplasia can be difficult. Reactive fibroblasts arising in granulation tissue are often pleomorphic and can be easily mistaken for malignant neoplastic cells.
- The Vaccine Associated Feline Sarcoma Task Force (VAFSTF) recommends that every mass that: (i) persists for more than 3 months; (ii) is larger than 2 cm; and (iii) increases in size 1 month after injection should be biopsied (3-2-1 rule). Incisional biopsy is preferred to Tru-cut biopsy, since the tumour can be heterogeneous and can be misdiagnosed as a granuloma for small tissue samples. Given the highly infiltrative nature of this tumour, advanced imaging (CT scan) must be performed prior to surgical excision.

# Further reading

Martano, M., Morello, E. and Buracco, P. (2011) Feline injection-site sarcoma: past, present and future perspectives. *Veterinary Journal* 188, 136–141.

# Rhabdomyoma and rhabdomyosarcoma

Tumours of the skeletal muscle deriving from myofibroblasts or primitive mesenchymal cells capable of differentiation into skeletal muscle cells.

## Clinical features

- Very rare skin neoplasms in dogs and cats. The benign form is more rare than the malignant counterpart.
- No age, breed or sex predilection reported. However, several cases of rhabdomyosarcoma described in the literature have been observed in young dogs (< 2 years old).
- Rhabdomyoma has been primarily reported in the larynx and ear pinnae in dogs and cats, respectively. Rhabdomyosarcoma may be observed in several locations in both species. In cats, it may also develop at the site of previous injection or vaccination.
- Most tumours present as firm, poorly demarcated, often multilobulated masses, which arise in the underlying muscle. Alopecia and ulceration are common.
- Rhabdomyoma is a slow-growing tumour.
- Rhabdomyosarcoma is characterized by a more aggressive behaviour and metastatic potential.

## Cytological features

- Variable cytological features, often non-specific.
- The cellularity is variable, from low to high.
- Background: clear and variably haemodiluted.
- Cell morphology greatly depends on the histological variant.
- They are often individualized, round to polygonal and with a low N:C ratio. Additional populations of elongated cells and smaller cells with a high N:C ratio can also be seen (undifferentiated rhabdomyoblasts).
- Nuclei are round, central to paracentral. They have granular chromatin. Prominent round nucleoli are often visible in the malignant forms.
- Cytoplasm is abundant, basophilic, often granular, with poorly defined borders. Cytoplasmic cross-striation and paranuclear clear halo may be seen occasionally.
- Cellularity and cellular atypia are higher in malignant forms and may include marked anisocytosis/anisokaryosis, multinucleation and bizarre mitotic figures. Multinucleated cells may have nuclei arranged in a linear fashion within the cytoplasm (strap cells).

## Variants

Four different histological variants of rhabdomyosarcoma have been reported in the literature and include botryoid, embryonal, alveolar and pleomorphic forms. The botryoid types mainly affect the urinary bladder, whereas the other forms have been described originating from striated muscle of the outer body surface.

- Embryonal rhabdomyosarcoma:
  - This is the most common variant and has been reported in dogs and only rarely in cats.
  - Head and neck are preferred anatomical locations.
  - Cells may exhibit different stages of development from round to polygonal and often show marked signs of atypia.
  - A spindle-cell sub-variant has also been described in literature.

- Alveolar rhabdomyosarcoma:
  - Uncommon form, mostly observed in young dogs.
  - It presents as mass lesion in various sites.
  - Cells may be individualized or forming poorly cohesive groups.
  - Aspirates exfoliate variable numbers of round to oval cells with a high N:C ratio and variably defined margins. The cytoplasm is scant to moderate and can contain small clear punctate vacuoles.
  - Occasionally, the individual cell morphology may resemble large lymphoid cells.
  - Anisokaryosis and anisocytosis are moderate.
  - Mitotic figures can be frequent.
- Pleomorphic rhabdomyosarcoma:
  - Very uncommon form, only rarely reported in dogs and cats and mostly in the larger muscles of the limbs.
  - In practice, it can be difficult to differentiate pleomorphic rhabdomyosarcoma from embryonal and alveolar types, as they may look similar. Cells often shown marked features of atypia.

> **Differential diagnoses**
> - Soft tissue sarcoma of other origin
> - Histiocytic sarcoma
> - Round cell tumour:
>   - Extramedullary plasmacytoma
>   - Lymphoma

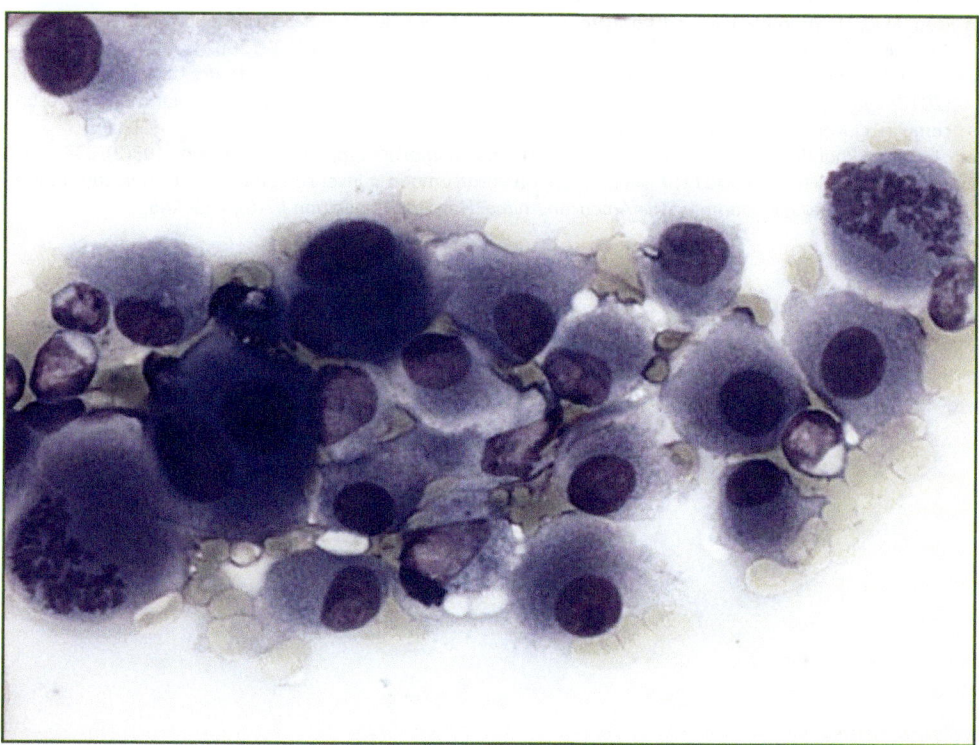

**Fig. 9.21.** Dog. Embryonal rhabdomyosarcoma. Wright-Giemsa. (*Courtesy of Giancarlo Avallone, University of Bologna, Italy.*)

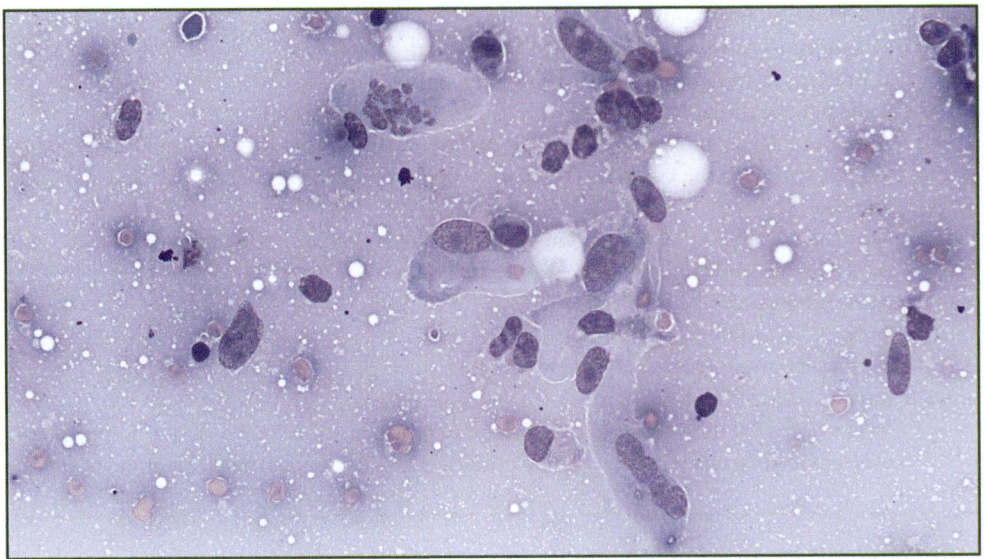

**Fig. 9.22.** Cat. Rhabdomyosarcoma. Note the marked cytological features of atypia and the presence of a strap cell. Wright-Giemsa.

## Further reading

Caserto, B.G. (2013) A comparative review of canine and human rhabdomyosarcoma with emphasis on classification and pathogenesis. *Veterinary Pathology* 55(5), 806–826.

Da Roza, M.R., De Amorim, R.F. and Carneiro, F.P. (2010) Aggressive spindle cell rhabdomyosarcoma in an 11-month-old boxer dog. *Journal of Veterinary Medical Science* 72(10), 1363–1366.

Murakami, M., Sakai, H., Iwatani, N., Asakura, A., Hoshino, Y., Mori, T., Yanai, T., Maruo, L.K. and Masegi, T. (2010) Cytologic, histologic, and immunohistochemical features of maxillofacial alveolar rhabdomyosarcoma in a juvenile dog. *Veterinary Clinical Pathology* 39(1), 113–118.

Roth, L. (1990) Rhabdomyoma of the ear pinna in four cats. *Journal of Comparative Pathology* 103(2), 237–240.

Snyder, L.A. and Michael, H. (2011) Alveolar rhabdomyosarcoma in a juvenile Labrador Retriever: case report and literature review. *Journal of the American Animal Hospital Association* 47(6), 443–446.

# 9.2 Histiocytic Tumours

## Histiocytic sarcoma (HS)

Malignant tumour of histiocytic origin deriving from interstitial dendritic cells (DCs).

### Clinical features

- Most commonly described in dogs, very rare in cats.
- Localized forms are reported in several organs, including the skin.
- The disease is considered disseminated when it spreads beyond the local draining lymph node and involves distant sites. This disease was previously known as malignant histiocytosis.
- Solitary or multiple, variably sized, cutaneous or subcutaneous masses. In dogs, most tumour masses are located on extremities, especially in the periarticular regions (e.g. elbow and stifle); in cats, they have been reported on the extremities and abdomen.
- Localized histiocytic sarcoma has a better prognosis than the disseminated form, if treated early with wide surgical excision. The prognosis of the disseminated form is poor.
- Over-represented canine breeds: Bernese Mountain Dog, Rottweiler, Golden Retriever, Flat-coated Retriever and Miniature Schnauzer.

### Cytological features

- Cellularity is variable, often high.
- Background: clear to lightly basophilic and variably haemodiluted.
- Neoplastic cells are pleomorphic. They are usually round to oval, slightly elongated and occasionally with small cytoplasmic tails. They exfoliate individually.
- Nuclei are round to oval, often large, with coarse, granular or clumped chromatin. They are eccentric to paracentral. Multiple prominent and irregularly shaped nucleoli are frequently seen.
- The cytoplasm is lightly or occasionally moderately basophilic, and moderate in amount. It may contain clear intracytoplasmic vacuoles or small phagosomes.
- Neoplastic cells can display erythrophagocytosis.
- Cytological features of atypia are often but not always prominent. Anisocytosis and anisokaryosis are variable to marked and the N:C ratio is variable. Binucleation and/or multinucleation and frequent mitotic figures are often seen. In some cases, the pleomorphism is less prominent and anisokaryosis and anisocytosis are modest.

**Differential diagnoses**
- Soft tissue sarcoma
- Anaplastic sarcoma of giant cells
- Synovial sarcoma (for articular histiocytic sarcoma)
- Osteosarcoma

**Pearls and Pitfalls**

Cytology is often diagnostic. However, in less straightforward cases, a definitive diagnosis may require histopathology and immunohistochemistry. The most specific marker used on formalin-fixed samples is the ionized calcium-binding adaptor molecule 1 (IBA1).

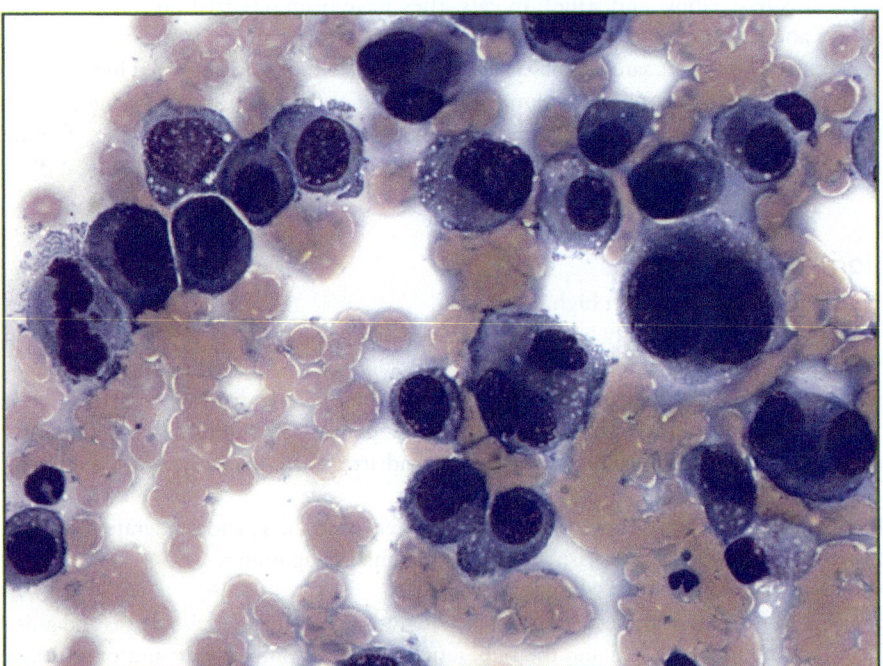

**Fig. 9.23.** Dog. Histiocytic sarcoma. Neoplastic cells show marked anisokaryosis, binucleation and atypical mitoses. Wright-Giemsa.

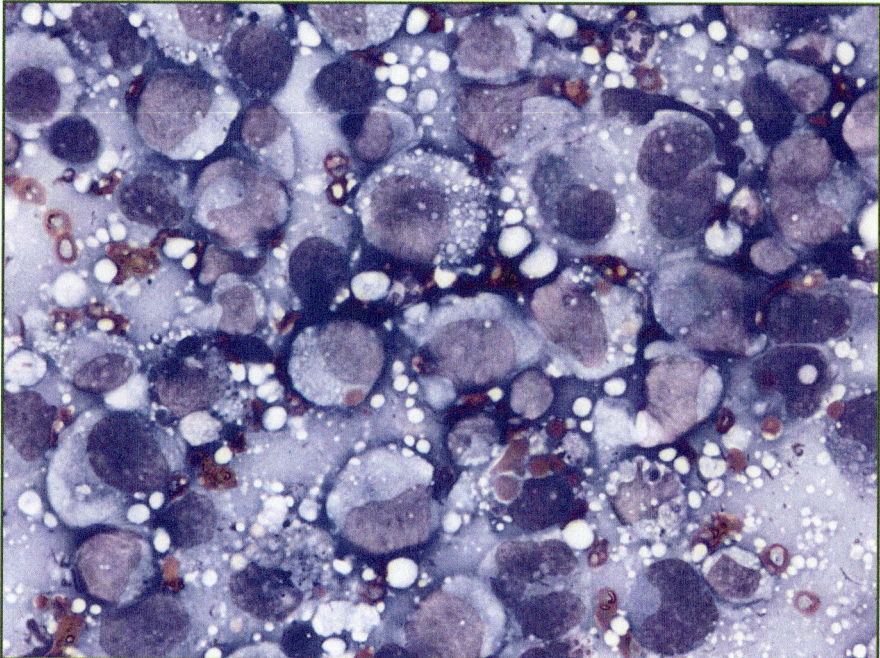

**Fig. 9.24.** Dog. Histiocytic sarcoma. Neoplastic cells are vacuolated and show features of atypia. Wright-Giemsa.

## Further reading

Lenz, J.A., Furrow, E., Craig, L.E. and Cannon, C.M. (2017) Histiocytic sarcoma in 14 miniature schnauzers – a new breed predisposition? *Journal of Small Animal Practice* 58(8), 461–467.
Moore, P.F. (2014) A review of histiocytic diseases of dogs and cats, *Veterinary Pathology* 51(1), 167–184.

# Feline progressive dendritic cell histiocytosis (FPH)

Histiocytic disease arising from interstitial dendritic cells.

## Clinical features
- Disease of middle-aged to older cats (7–17 years).
- Presenting either as a solitary skin nodule or multiple papules, nodules or plaques. Lesions measure up to 1.5 cm in diameter; they are firm, often alopecic, non-pruritic and non-painful. They may wax and wane, but spontaneous regression does not occur. Involvement of lymph nodes and internal organs can be observed.
- Preferred locations include the head, lower extremities and trunk.
- The initial clinical course is indolent and the neoplasm behaves like a low-grade disease. However, long-term prognosis is poor, as the disease is progressive.

## Cytological features
- The cellularity is variable, from low to high.
- Background: clear to lightly basophilic, variably haemodiluted.
- Neoplastic cells are round to polygonal, rarely spindloid, with poorly defined cytoplasmic borders. They exfoliate either individually or in poorly cohesive groups.
- Nuclei are oval to reniform, occasionally indented, paracentral to eccentric, with finely stippled to reticular chromatin. A single, round and prominent nucleolus is occasionally visible.
- The cytoplasm is moderate to abundant and lightly basophilic. It may contain rare clear vacuoles and, at times, it may appear wispy and paler at the outer edges.
- Anisocytosis and anisokaryosis are variable, generally moderate to marked. Binucleation, multinucleation and rare mitotic figures can be found.
- Low numbers of small lymphocytes, mast cells and other inflammatory cells are not uncommon.

### Pearls and Pitfalls
Presumptive diagnosis can be attempted by assessment of the cytomorphology in conjunction with the clinical presentation. Definitive confirmation of the dendritic lineage requires immunophenotyping and this can be obtained specifically by demonstrating CD1 expression on cytological or histological preparations.

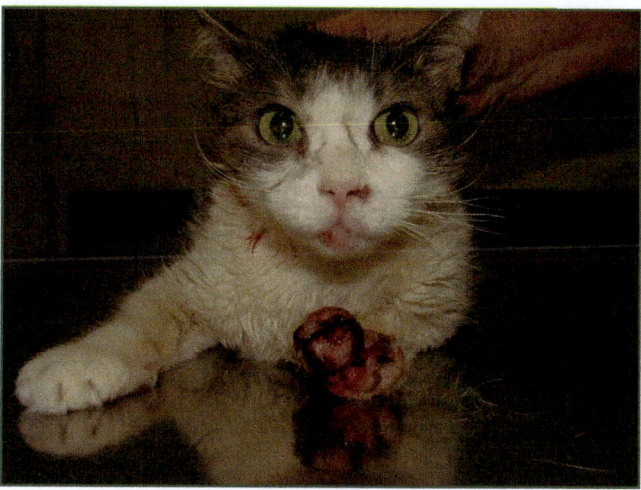

**Fig. 9.25.** Cat. Feline progressive dendritic cell histiocytosis. (*Courtesy of Fabrizio Fabbrini, Clinica Veterinaria Papiniano, Italy.*)

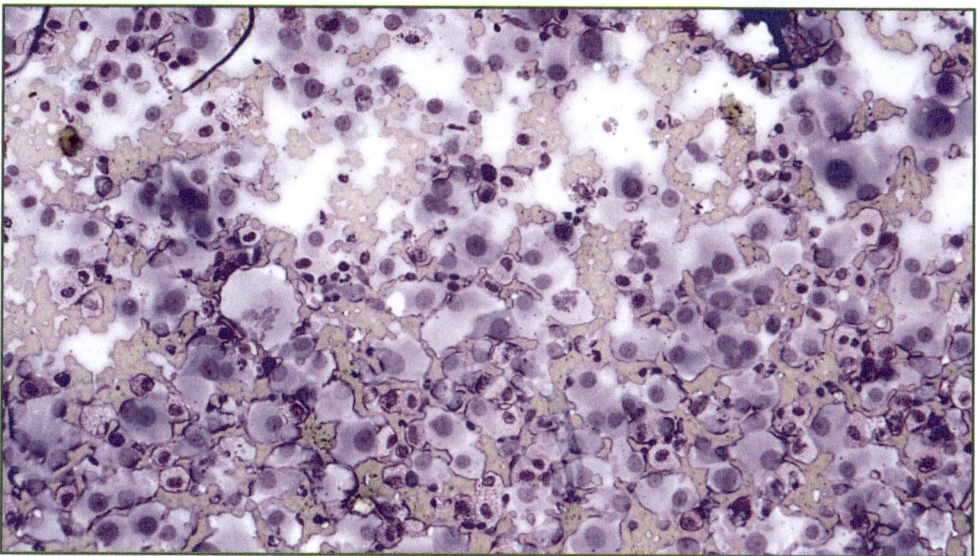

**Fig. 9.26.** Cat. Feline progressive dendritic cell histiocytosis. Neoplastic cells appear polygonal and show marked cytological features of atypia. Wright-Giemsa. (*Courtesy of Alice Pastorello, DWR Diagnostics, UK.*)

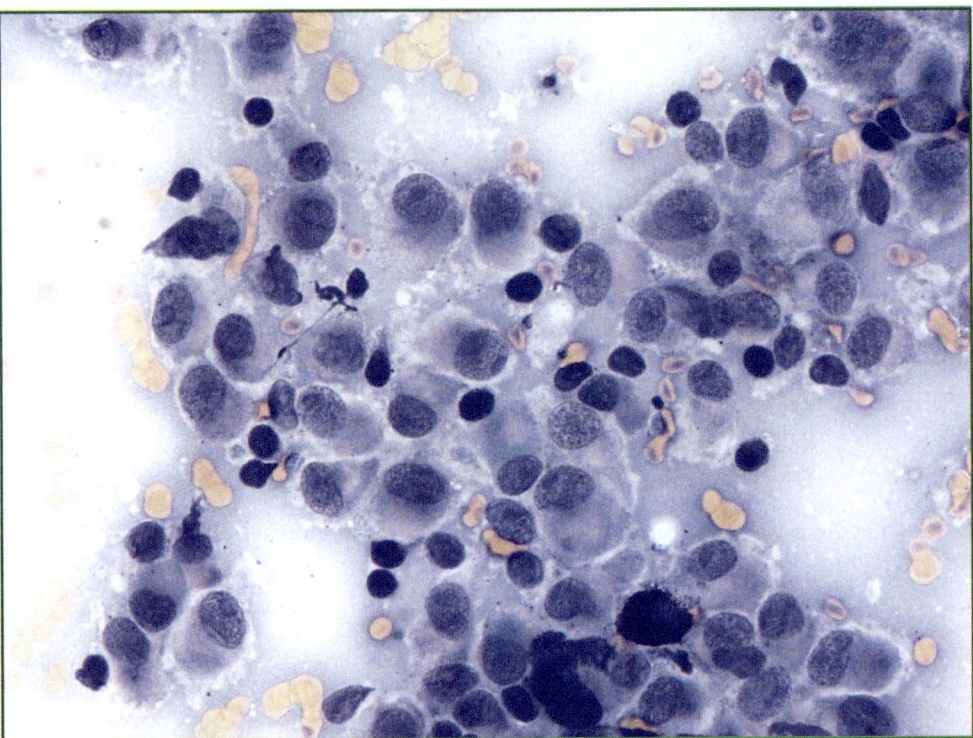

**Fig. 9.27.** Cat. Feline progressive dendritic cell histiocytosis. Amongst neoplastic cells there are scattered granulated mast cells and small lymphocytes. Wright-Giemsa.

## Further reading

Moore, P.F. (2014) A review of histiocytic diseases of dogs and cats. *Veterinary Pathology* 51(1), 167–184.
Pinto da Cunha, N., Ghisleni, G., Scarampella, F., Fabbrini, F., Sforna, M., Cornegliani, L., Caniatti, M., Avallone, G., Moore, P. and Roccabianca, P. (2014) Cytologic and immunocytochemical characterization of feline progressive histiocytosis. *Veterinary Clinical Pathology* 43(3), 428–436.

# Other canine histiocytic disorders

Cutaneous Langerhans cell histiocytosis (LCH) and (reactive) cutaneous histiocytosis (CH).

## Clinical features

- Canine cutaneous Langerhans cell histiocytosis (LCH):
  - Largely benign tumour of histiocytic origin, deriving from Langherans cells (LCs).
  - Multiple lesions (up to several hundred) ranging from nodules to masses, which may undergo spontaneous regression or may extend and ulcerate in approximately 50% of the cases.
  - Involvement of lymph nodes and internal organs may occur. This is associated with poor prognosis.
  - Over-represented canine breed: Shar Pei.
- Canine cutaneous (reactive) histiocytosis (CH):
  - Histiocytic inflammatory disease deriving from the interstitial dendritic cells and causing, together with T-lymphocytes, a lympho-histiocytic vasculitis. When involving lymph nodes and other organs, it is defined as systemic histiocytosis (SH).
  - Multiple cutaneous and subcutaneous nodules, often ulcerated. Head, face, trunk, scrotum, nose and extremities are considered preferred locations. New lesions may appear at different sites.
  - Spontaneous regression is common.

## Cytological features

- Canine cutaneous Langerhans cell histiocytosis:
  - Histiocytic cells are similar to those observed in histiocytoma.
  - Anisokaryosis may be more prominent than in histiocytoma and multinucleation can be present, especially in clinically aggressive cases. However, this is not a consistent feature.
- Canine cutaneous (reactive) histiocytosis:
  - Aspirates yield a mixed cell population with prevalence of histiocytes and small lymphocytes. Histiocytes lack cytological atypia.
  - Variable percentages of neutrophils, plasma cells and eosinophils may also be observed.

### Differential diagnoses

- Canine cutaneous Langerhans cell histiocytosis (LCH):
  - Cutaneous histiocytoma (when multiple lesions are present)
- Canine cutaneous (reactive) histiocytosis:
  - Mixed (chronic) inflammation
  - Inflamed cutaneous lymphoma

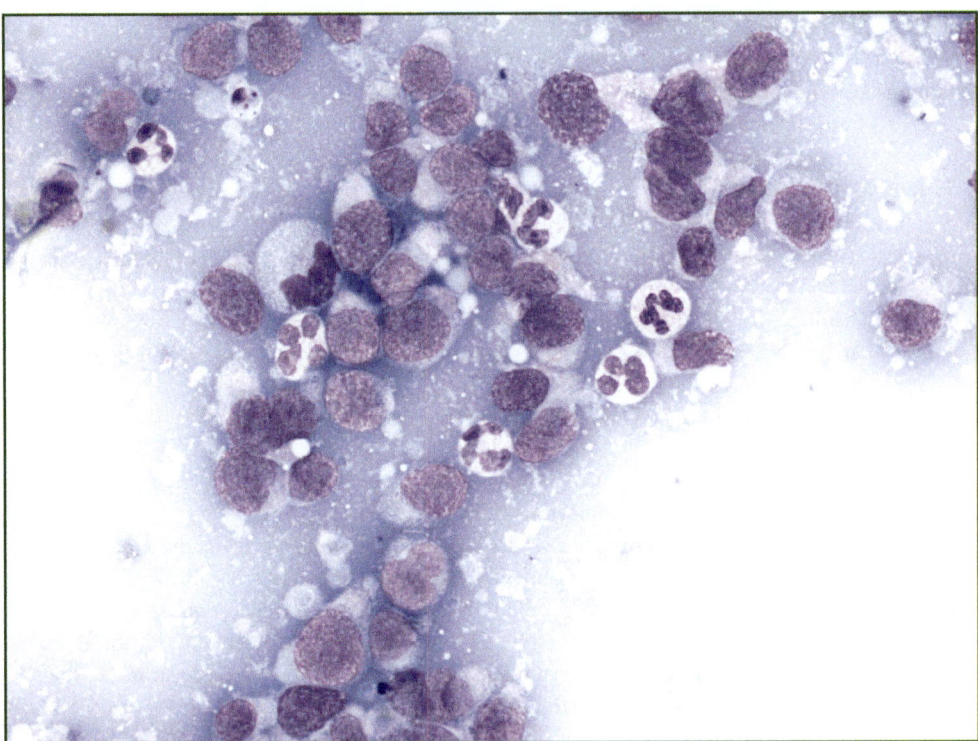

**Fig. 9.28.** Dog. Cutaneous Langerhans cell histiocytosis. Histiocytes show cytological features of atypia, which are more prominent than in cutaneous histiocytoma. Wright-Giemsa.

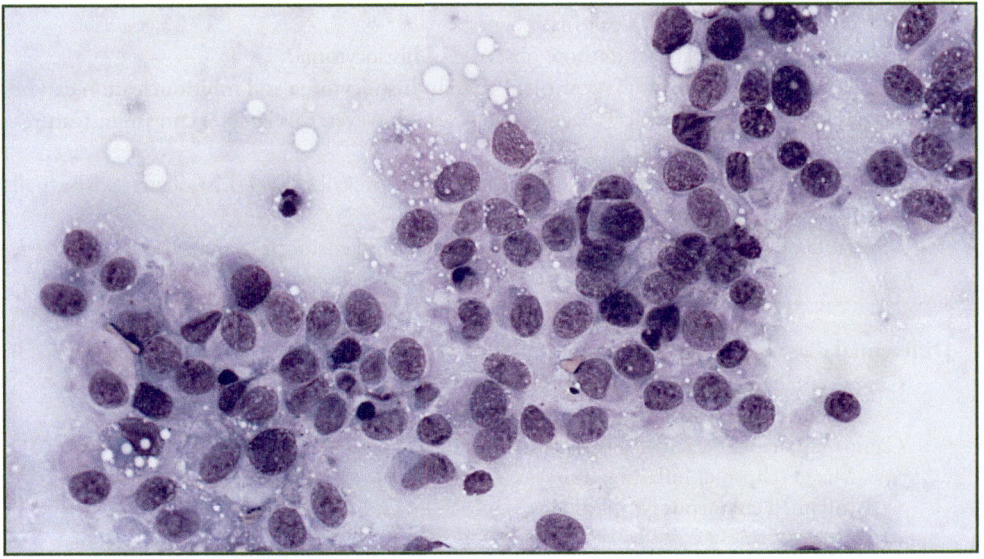

**Fig. 9.29.** Dog. Cutaneous Langherans cell histiocytosis. Wright-Giemsa. (*Courtesy of Nic Ilchyshyn, DWR Diagnostics, UK.*)

**Table 9.1.** Histiocytic diseases of dogs affecting the skin and subcutis.

| | Cell of origin | Key clinical features | Key cytological features | Immunophenotype |
|---|---|---|---|---|
| Histiocytoma | Langerhans cells | • Solitary, dome-shaped, exophytic, often red, cutaneous masses, often alopecic and/or ulcerated<br>• Benign clinical behaviour, regression often observed | • Histiocytes<br>• Small lymphocytes (during the regression phase) | CD1a, CD11c/ CD18, E-cadherin, IBA1 |
| Cutaneous Langerhans cell histiocytosis (LCH) | Langerhans cells | • Multiple cutaneous nodules, which may either regress or become coalescent and ulcerate<br>• Largely benign process, involvement of lymph nodes and internal organs is uncommon and is associated with poorer prognosis | • Histiocytes<br>• Morphology similar to histiocytoma. Anisokaryosis and anisocytosis can be more pronounced and multinucleation may be observed | CD1a, CD11c/ CD18, E-cadherin, IBA1 |
| Cutaneous (reactive) histiocytosis (CH) | Interstitial dendritic cells | • Multiple cutaneous and subcutaneous nodules, often ulcerated. When disseminated, it is referred to as systemic histiocytosis (SH)<br>• Spontaneous regression is common | • Mixed cell population<br>• Prevalence of histiocytes and small lymphocytes<br>• Other inflammatory cells may be present | CD1a, CD4, CD11c/ CD18, CD90, IBA1 |
| Histiocytic sarcoma (HS) | Interstitial dendritic cells | • Solitary or multiple subcutaneous masses. When involving distant sites it is referred to as disseminated histiocytic sarcoma<br>• Prognosis is poor especially in the disseminated form | • Pleomorphic population of discrete to slightly spindloid cells with variable features of atypia | CD1a, CD11c/ CD18, IBA1 |

# Further reading

Moore, P.F. (2014) A review of histiocytic diseases of dogs and cats. *Veterinary Pathology* 51(1), 167–184.

## 9.3 Melanocytic Tumours

Group of tumours arising from the melanocytes in the epidermis, dermis, or adnexa.

### Clinical features
- Common neoplasms in dogs (5% of all skin tumours); less often observed in cats (3%).
- They include a benign (*melanocytoma*) and malignant (*melanoma*) form, the latter representing 19% and 33% of the total cutaneous melanocytic tumours in the dog and cat, respectively.
- Age:
  - Dogs: 7–12 years (melanocytoma), 10–13 years (melanoma).
  - Cats: 4–13 years (melanocytoma), 8–12 (melanoma).
- Melanocytic tumours appear as variably sized and variably pigmented, circumscribed, raised cutaneous lesions. They are often alopecic and may be ulcerated, inflamed and infiltrative, especially when malignant.
- Anatomical sites:
  - Dogs: head (especially eyelid) and trunk for melanocytoma. Melanoma frequently arises from the oral cavity, mucucutaneous junctions and nail bed.
  - Cats: head (including pinnae, lips and nose) and back for both melanocytoma and melanoma.
- The majority of melanocytomas in dogs are slow-growing masses. Surgical excision is curative.
- Melanomas are often rapidly growing and can be fatal. Metastases usually occur to the draining lymph nodes, lung and occasionally to other internal organs.
- Over-represented canine breeds:
  - Melanocytoma: Hungarian Vizsla, Miniature Schnauzer, Irish Setter, Schnauzer and Australian Terrier.
  - Melanoma: Schnauzer, Miniature Schnauzer, Giant Schnauzer, Chow Chow, Shar Pei and Scottish Terrier.

### Cytological features
- Cellularity is variable. Often medium-high especially in malignant forms.
- Background: variably haemodiluted, may contain free melanin granules.
- The aspirates are composed of nucleated cells that contain variable numbers of fine black-green round or rice-shaped granules of melanin.
- Cells exfoliate singly, in cohesive clusters or in aggregates. They range from round to stellate to spindloid in both benign and malignant forms.
- Nuclei are round to oval, central to paracentral. In melanocytomas, nuclei are often obscured by the intracytoplasmic melanin granules. The chromatin is finely stippled to coarse. In melanomas, the chromatin is often clumped and nucleoli are usually prominent, multiple and variably shaped.

- The cytoplasm is moderate in amount, basophilic and contains variable numbers of melanin granules; these may be few or absent in poorly differentiated (amelanotic) forms.
- Anisocytosis, anisokaryosis and atypical mitotic figures are often seen in melanomas.
- Melanin-laden macrophages (melanophages) are often seen. They can be difficult to differentiate from the melanocytes.

## Variants

Several histopathological variants of melanomas have been described in dogs and cats. These variants do not carry any prognostic significance; however, the epithelioid type of malignant melanoma in the cat may behave in a more aggressive and malignant fashion. The balloon cell variant has a characteristic appearance.

- Balloon cell variant:
  - Rare variant. Also called clear cell melanoma.
  - Cytologically, it is characterized by a population of large, round to polygonal cells with abundant clear or pale basophilic cytoplasm containing clear intracytoplasmic vacuoles. Cytological features of atypia can be marked.

**Differential diagnoses**
- Melanocytoma:
  - Melanoma
  - Pigmented trichoblastoma and basal cell tumour (especially in cats)
  - Sweat gland adenoma (may contain melanin)
- Melanoma:
  - Melanocytoma
  - Soft tissue sarcoma (for spindle cell variant only)
  - Histiocytic sarcoma (for amelanotic form only)
  - Sebaceous cell carcinoma, liposarcoma, clear cell adnexal carcinoma (for balloon cell variant only)

**Pearls and Pitfalls**
- In dogs, as a general rule, melanocytic neoplasms arising from the haired skin are most frequently benign, whereas those arising from nail beds, mucucutaneous junctions and oral mucosa are more commonly malignant.
- When undertaking cytological examination of regional lymph nodes for metastasis, care must be taken to differentiate melanophages from neoplastic melanocytes.
- For the diagnosis of amelanotic and poorly melanotic melanomas, special cytochemical (e.g. Fontana-Masson) or immunohistochemical (e.g. Melan A) stains can aid in the diagnostic process.

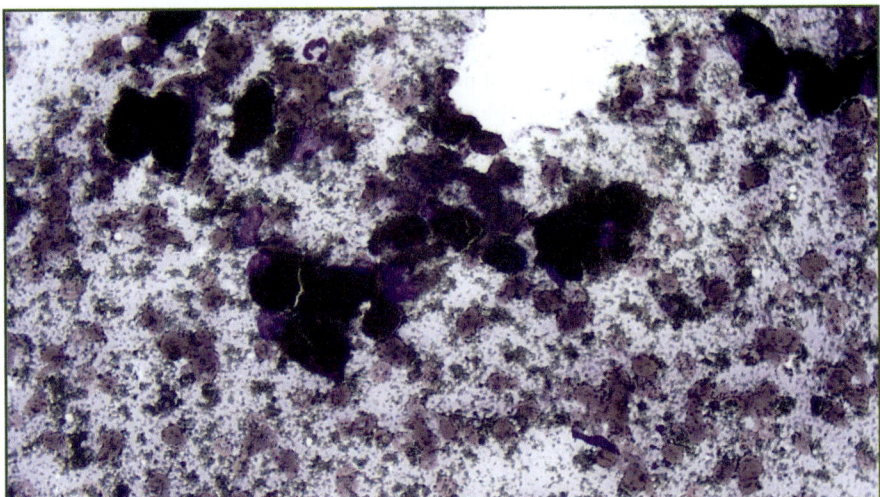

**Fig. 9.30.** Dog. Melanocytoma. Wright-Giemsa.

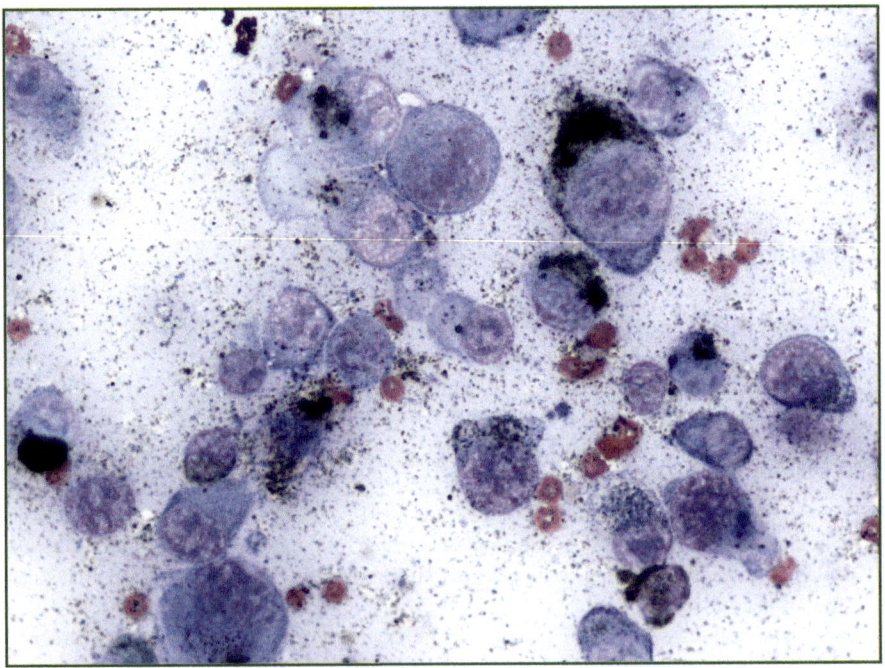

**Fig. 9.31.** Dog. Melanoma. Wright-Giemsa.

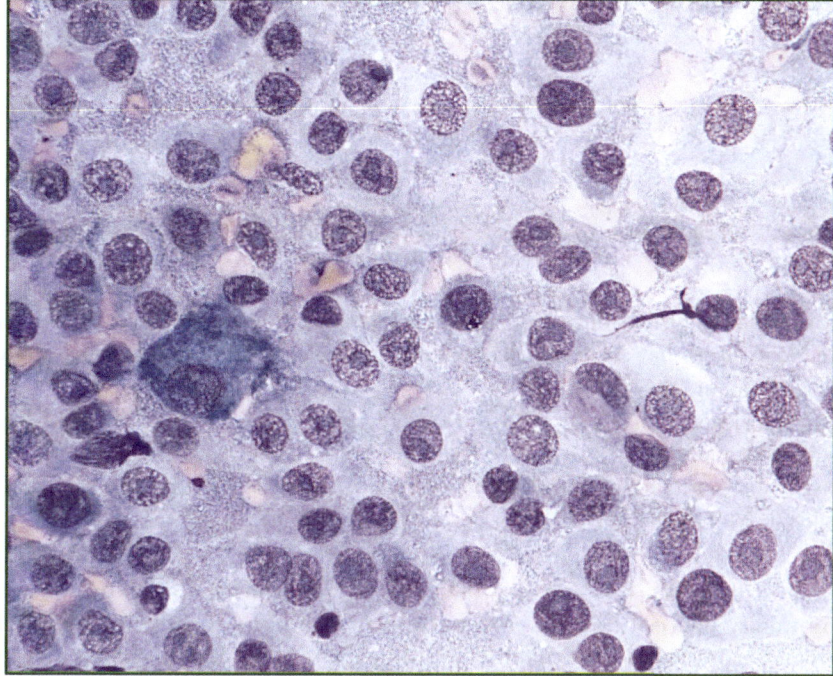

**Fig. 9.32.** Dog. Amelanotic melanoma. Most neoplastic cells do not contain melanin granules. Cytological features of atypia are moderate, including prominent nucleoli. Wright-Giemsa.

## Further reading

Van Der Linde Sipman, J.S., De Witt, M.M., Van Garderen, E., Molenbeek, R.F., Velde Zimmermann, D. and De Weger, R.A. (1997) Cutaneous malignant melanomas in 57 cats: identification of (amelanotic) signet-ring and balloon cell types and verification of their origin by immunohistochemistry, electron microscopy, and in situ hybridization. *Veterinary Pathology* 34(1), 31–38.

Wilkerson, M.J., Dolce, K., DeBey, B.M., Heeb, H. and Davidson, H. (2003) Metastatic balloon cell melanoma in a dog. *Veterinary Clinical Pathology* 32(1), 31–36.

# 10 Round Cell Tumours

Neoplasms included in this group originate from different cell lines, but have been historically grouped all together as they share similar cytological features. Round cell tumours include:

- Mast cell tumour (MCT).
- Cutaneous histiocytoma.
- Plasma cell tumour.
- Transmissible venereal tumour (TVT).
- Cutaneous lymphoma.

## Cytological diagnosis of cutaneous round cell tumours

Aspiration from round cell tumours usually harvests high numbers of cells. These cells are discrete, round to oval shaped, hence the name. Although round cells do not cluster together or produce extracellular matrix, in very thick and hypercellular aspirates they may give the impression of forming organized structures. In this case, it is important to look at their arrangement in the thinnest areas of the slides.

Each of the round cell tumours listed above has additional specific morphological features that facilitate their recognition on cytology. The ability to differentiate cytologically different round cell tumours is clinically important, as the biological behaviour of these neoplasms and the therapeutic options differ significantly. As an example, cutaneous histiocytoma often undergoes spontaneous regression, whereas mast cell tumour is generally approached with wide surgical excision and may have malignant potential. The morphology of these tumours will be described in detail in this chapter.

# 10.1 Canine Mast Cell Tumour (Canine MCT)

Neoplasia of mast cells.

## Clinical features

- Common neoplasm of the dog, accounting for approximately 21% of canine skin tumours.
- Age: mostly occurs in adult and old animals, with an average of approximately 9 years. However, it can be observed in dogs of any age, including puppies.
- Cutaneous mast cell tumour (MCT) is the most common form, followed by subcutaneous MCT. The differentiation between the two is based on clinical and histological examination.
    - Cutaneous MCT: can develop anywhere in the body. Macroscopically, it ranges from nodular rashes to diffuse swellings or, most commonly, hairless raised erythematous solid lesions. Masses can be ulcerated. Multiple forms can also occur, especially in Boxer, Boston Terrier, Golden Retriever and Pug.
    - Subcutaneous MCT: arises in the subcutaneous adipose tissue and presents as soft, fleshy masses. Legs, back and thorax are the most common sites.
- Variable biological behaviour: this mostly depends on histological grading (for cutaneous MCT), proliferation indexes (e.g. Ki67), c-Kit mutation and Kit receptor expression. High-grade cutaneous MCTs have an aggressive behaviour, with metastases starting from regional lymph nodes and often progressing to the spleen and liver in advanced stages. Peripheral blood involvement may also occur (mastocytaemia).
- MCTs in the oral mucosa or muzzle usually are more aggressive.
- As a general rule, subcutaneous MCTs tend to be less aggressive than cutaneous forms.
- Local and/or systemic paraneoplastic signs may be observed and are linked to the release of histamine, heparin and proteases contained within the mast cell granules. Local signs include oedema, ulceration and swelling at the primary tumour site, and possibly delayed wound healing and local coagulation abnormalities. The most common systemic effects are gastrointestinal signs and include vomiting, GI haemorrhage, anorexia and abdominal pain. Acute anaphylactic reactions are rare.
- Over-represented canine breeds: Boxer, Labrador Retriever, Golden Retriever, Shar Pei, Bulldog, Boston Terrier, Staffordshire Bull Terrier, Fox Terriers, Weimaraner, Cocker Spaniel, Rhodesian Ridgeback, Dachshund, Australian Cattle Dog, Beagle, Schnauzer and Pug.

## Cytological features

- Cellularity is variable, often high.
- Background: often clear, variably haemodiluted and with free purple granules from disrupted mast cells. It may contain collagen fibrils.
- Cells are round with a moderate N:C ratio.
- Nuclei are often obscured by the granules, especially in well-differentiated forms. When visible, they are medium sized, round to oval, mostly paracentral, with uniform to slightly clumped chromatin and variably visible nucleoli.

- The cytoplasm is moderate in amount and clear to pale basophilic. Rarely, an increased basophilia can be observed in high-grade tumours.
  - In well granulated forms, the cytoplasm contains numerous thick purple granules, usually evenly distributed within the cell.
  - In poorly granulated forms, granules are reduced in numbers and are usually finer. In these cases they may be polarized to one side of the nucleus or may form clumps.
- Occasionally, neoplastic cells can display erythrophagia.
- Cytological features of atypia are prominent in high-grade forms. These include karyomegaly, variable anisokaryosis and anisocytosis, bi- and/or multinucleation. Mitotic figures can be observed.
- A concurrent eosinophilic inflammation is often present. Eosinophils are attracted by the chemokines contained in the mast cell granules.
- Reactive fibroblasts are frequently seen. They may exhibit variable cytological pleomorphism and may contain eosinophilic/pink granules.
- Collagen fibrils may also be present.

---

**Differential diagnoses**
- Mast cell rich inflammatory lesion (e.g. insect bite reaction)
- Round cell tumour of other origin (in poorly granulated forms or Diff-Quik slides)

---

**Pearls and Pitfalls**
- Histopathology is always required to differentiate between cutaneous and subcutaneous forms and, in the case of a cutaneous MCT, for histopathological grading, which has been reported to have a prognostic significance. The most widely used grading systems are the three-tier Patnaik and the two-tier Kiupel systems. Nowadays, most anatomical pathologists apply both grading systems to all canine cutaneous mast cell tumours. The Patnaik system designates MCTs as grade I (low), II (intermediate), or III (high), based on depth of invasion, cell and nuclear morphology and mitotic count. The Kiupel system designates MCTs as low-grade or high-grade based on mitotic count, presence of multinucleation, bizarre nuclei and karyomegaly.
- As discussed above, the accurate grading of MCTs remains pertinent to the histopathology. However, based on a study by Camus *et al.* (2016), a cutaneous MCT is defined as high-grade on cytology when cells are either poorly granulated or when at least two of the four following findings are observed: (i) mitotic figures; (ii) binucleated or multinucleated cells; (iii) nuclear pleomorphism; and (iv) > 50% anisokaryosis. Claimed sensitivity and specificity of this cytological grading scheme are 88% and 94%, respectively.
- Certain Romanowsky-type dyes (e.g. Diff-Quik) sometimes fail to stain mast cell granules. However, also in these cases, it should always be possible to find a few intracytoplasmic granules in some of the cells upon careful observation of the slide.

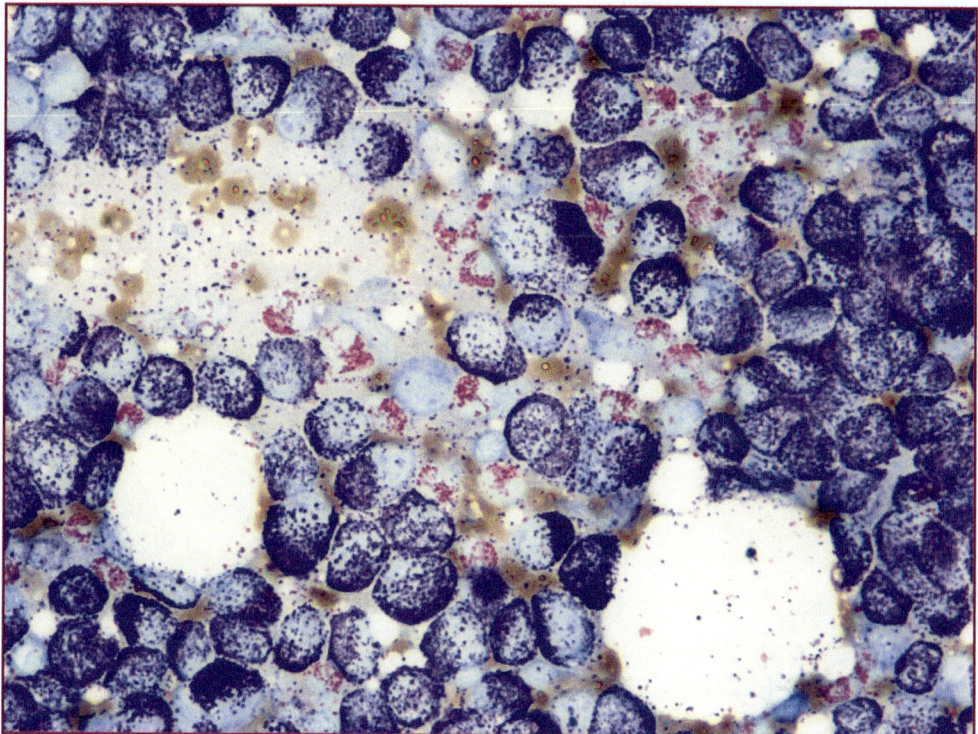

**Fig. 10.1.** Dog. Mast cell tumour. Granulated mast cells and eosinophils. Wright-Giemsa.

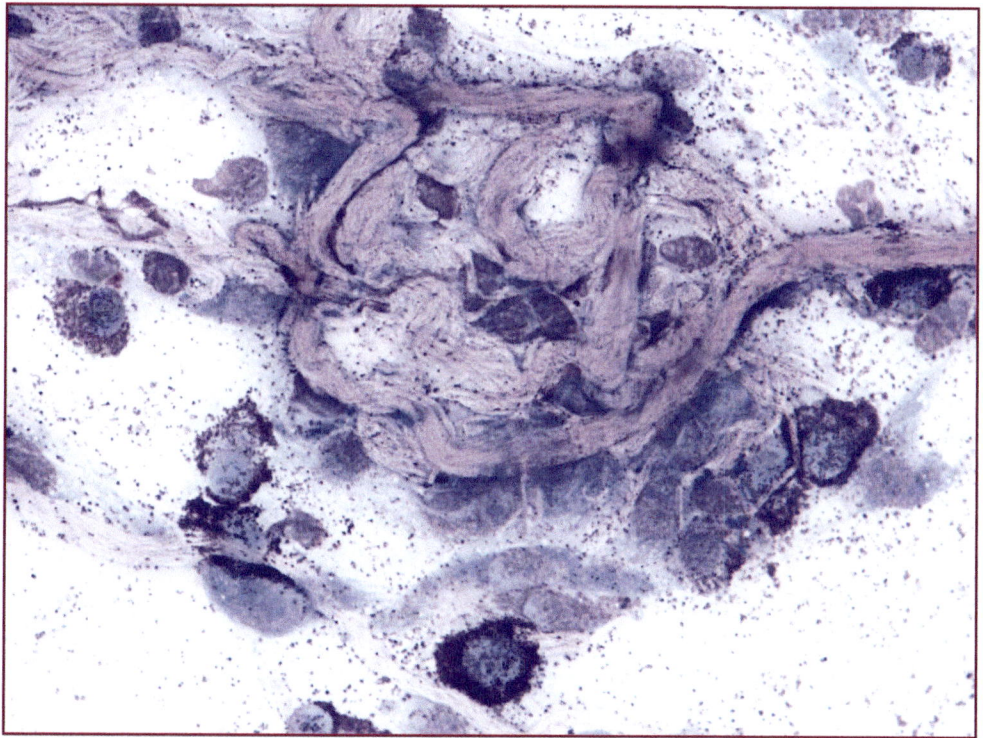

**Fig. 10.2.** Dog. Mast cell tumour. Mast cells admixed with ribbons of pink collagen fibrils and reactive fibroblasts. Wright-Giemsa.

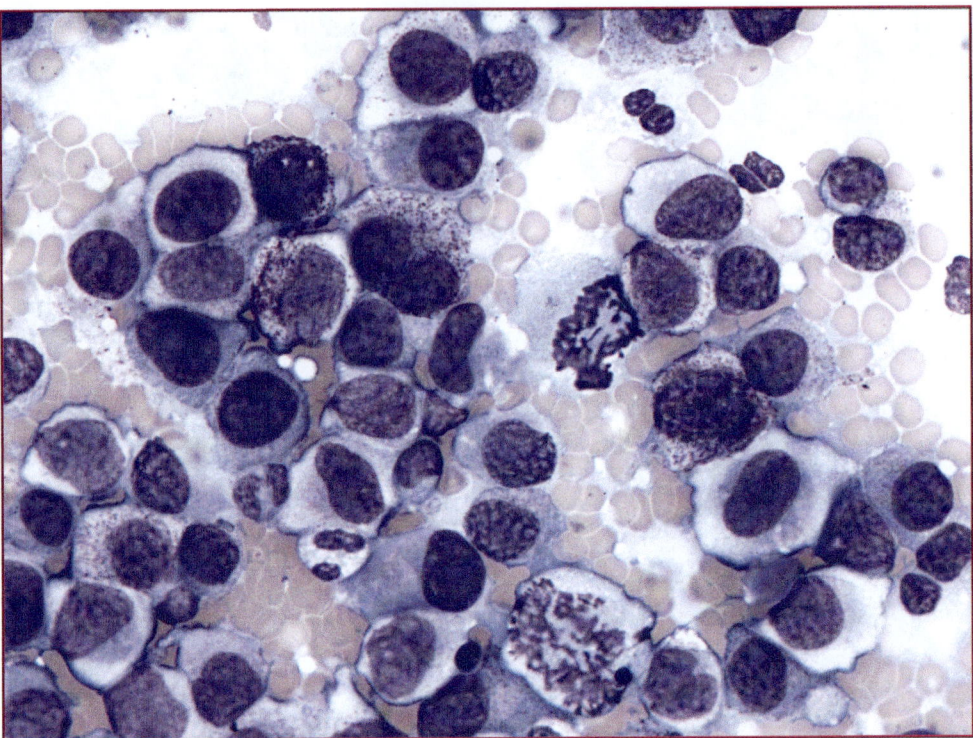

**Fig. 10.3.** Dog. Mast cell tumour. Mast cells are poorly granulated and show moderate anisokaryosis, binucleation and mitotic figures. Wright-Giemsa.

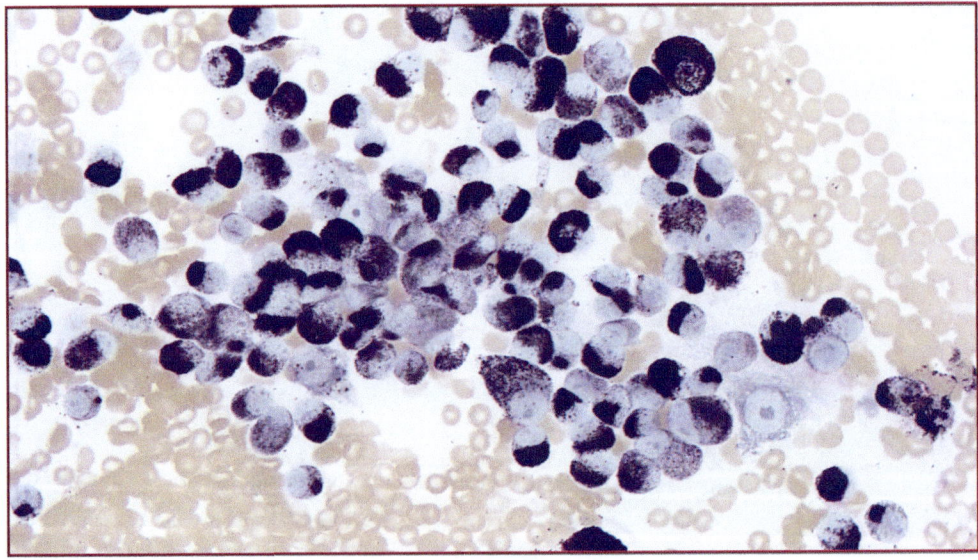

**Fig. 10.4.** Dog. Mast cell tumour. The granules are polarized to one side of the cells and occasionally clumped in small groups. Wright-Giemsa.

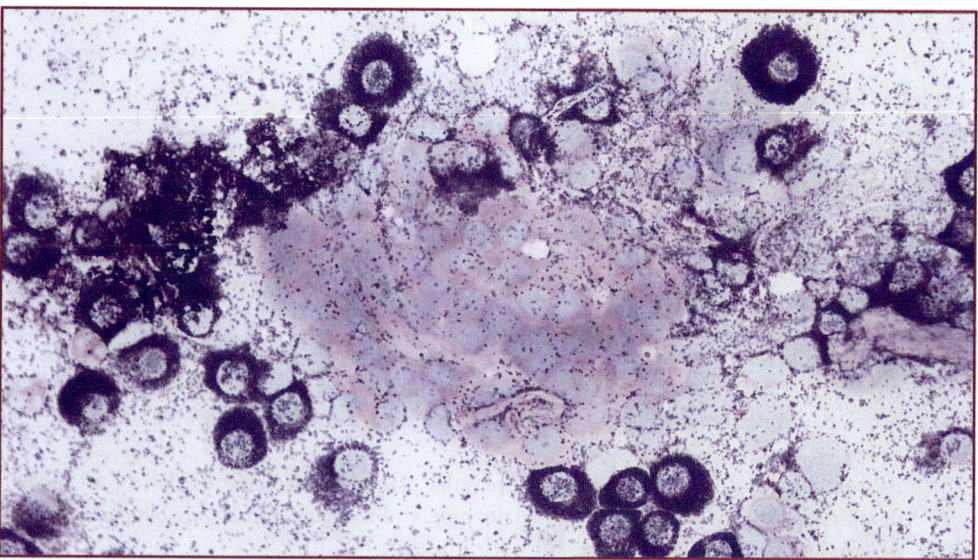

**Fig. 10.5.** Dog. Mast cell tumour. Cluster of poorly stained adnexal epithelial cells surrounded by granulated mast cells. Although uncommon, hyperplastic adnexal epithelial cells can exfoliate alongside the neoplastic mast cells. Wright-Giemsa.

# Reference and further reading

Blackwood, L., Murphy, S., Buracco, P., De Vos, J.P., De Fornel-Thibaud, P., Hirschberger, J., Kessler, M., Pastor, J., Ponce, P., Savary-Bataille, K. *et al.* (2012) European consensus document on mast cell tumours in dogs and cats. *Veterinary Comparative Oncology* 10(3), 1–29.

Camus, M.S., Priest, H.L and Koehler, J.W. (2016) Cytologic criteria for mast cell tumor grading in dogs with evaluation of clinical outcome. *Veterinary Pathology* 53(6), 117–1123.

Hergt, F., Von Bomhard, W. and Kent, S. (2016) Use of a 2-tier histologic grading system for canine cutaneous mast cell tumors on cytology specimens. *Veterinary Clinical Pathology*, 45(3), 477–483.

Scarpa, F., Sabattini, S. and Bettini, G. (2016) Cytological grading of canine cutaneous mast cell tumours. *Veterinary Comparative Oncology* 14(3), 245–251.

## 10.2   Feline Mast Cell Tumour (Feline MCT)

Neoplasia of mast cells.

### Clinical features

- Common neoplasm accounting for approximately 7% and 21% of all feline skin tumours, according to previous European and American studies, respectively. Visceral forms are much more common than in dogs and account for up to 50% of all feline mast cell tumours (MCTs).
- Age: adult cats are more frequently affected, with an average of approximately 10 years. However, it can be observed in cats of any age. No sex predisposition reported.
- It can develop anywhere in the body, with preference for head (especially in young animals), neck, trunk and legs.
- It usually presents as a single firm tan papule, plaque or discrete nodule in the skin or subcutis. Overlying epidermis is usually pink and alopecic, but it may be ulcerated. Approximately 20% of cats present with multiple lesions.
- Mastocytaemia is uncommon.
- Cutaneous mast cell tumour is generally a benign neoplasm in cats, but up to 22% of cases may show an aggressive behaviour.
- Over-represented feline breeds: Siamese, Burmese, Russian Blue, Ragdoll, Maine Coon, Oriental and Havana cat.

### Cytological features

- Cellularity is variable, often high.
- Background: often clear, variably haemodiluted. It often contains free purple granules derived from the disruption of the mast cells during the smearing.
- Neoplastic mast cells are round with a moderate N:C ratio.
- Nuclei are often obscured by the granules. When visible, they are round to oval, mostly paracentral, with uniform to slightly clumped chromatin and variably visible nucleoli.
- The cytoplasm is clear or lightly basophilic, moderate to abundant and commonly contains numerous fine purple/magenta granules. Granules are often finer than in dogs. In poorly granulated forms, granules may be present in very low numbers and/or may have a patchy distribution.
- Cytological pleomorphism is variable and is more prominent in the pleomorphic variant. Anisocytosis and anisokaryosis can be moderate to marked and binucleation and/or multinucleation are often observed. Mitotic figures can be seen in variable numbers.
- Occasionally, neoplastic cells can display erythrophagia.
- Eosinophils are also present, but with a lower frequency than in canine MCT. Low numbers of small lymphocytes can also be observed.
- Reactive fibroblasts and collagen fibrils are rarely present.

### Variants

Histologically, feline MCTs can be subclassified in different forms. In the literature, the terminology is not standardized and there is inconsistency between studies. The following is the classification of feline cutaneous MCTs suggested by Kiupel (2016) in the latest edition of Meuten's *Tumors in Domestic Animals*.

- Well-differentiated form:
  - Most common form of feline MCT.
  - Neoplastic cells show little pleomorphism and resemble normal mast cells.
  - Eosinophilic infiltrates are rare or absent.
  - Small lymphocytes are often found.
- Pleomorphic form:
  - Uncommon form of feline MCT.
  - As per name, the cellular pleomorphism in this form is often prominent. Cytomegalic cells can be seen and anisokaryosis and anisocytosis can be marked. Multinucleated cells and cells with bizarre nuclei are observed.
  - Cell pleomorphism and nuclear atypia do not seem to correlate with a malignant behaviour.
  - Numerous eosinophils are often present.
- Atypical (histiocytic) form:
  - Rare form of feline MCT.
  - Seen mostly in young cats as multiple nodular lesions.
  - Associated with a benign clinical course or spontaneous regression.
  - Siamese cats may be predisposed.
  - Cytologically, neoplastic mast cells resemble histiocytes. They are large, polygonal to round, with lightly basophilic cytoplasm lacking the typical intracytoplasmic granules. Nuclei are large, round, often indented and paracentral. Mitotic activity is low.
  - Small lymphocytes are frequently present.

---

**Differential diagnoses**
- Mast cell rich inflammatory lesions (e.g. insect bite reaction)
- Eosinophilic granuloma

---

**Pearls and Pitfalls**
- Cytoplasmic granules are not as easy to see as in canine MCTs, especially if slides are stained with Diff-Quik. Hence, when possible, Wright-Giemsa stain is preferable.
- Feline MCTs are often referred to as compact or diffuse, mainly depending on their degree of invasiveness into the deeper subcutis. The use of these terms has not been consistent in the previous literature.
- The cellular pleomorphism is not associated with the clinical behaviour of feline MCTs. The only confirmed prognostic factor for feline MCTs is the mitotic activity. It is still unclear if other variables such as tumour diameter, presentation with multiple masses and histological parameters have a prognostic significance.

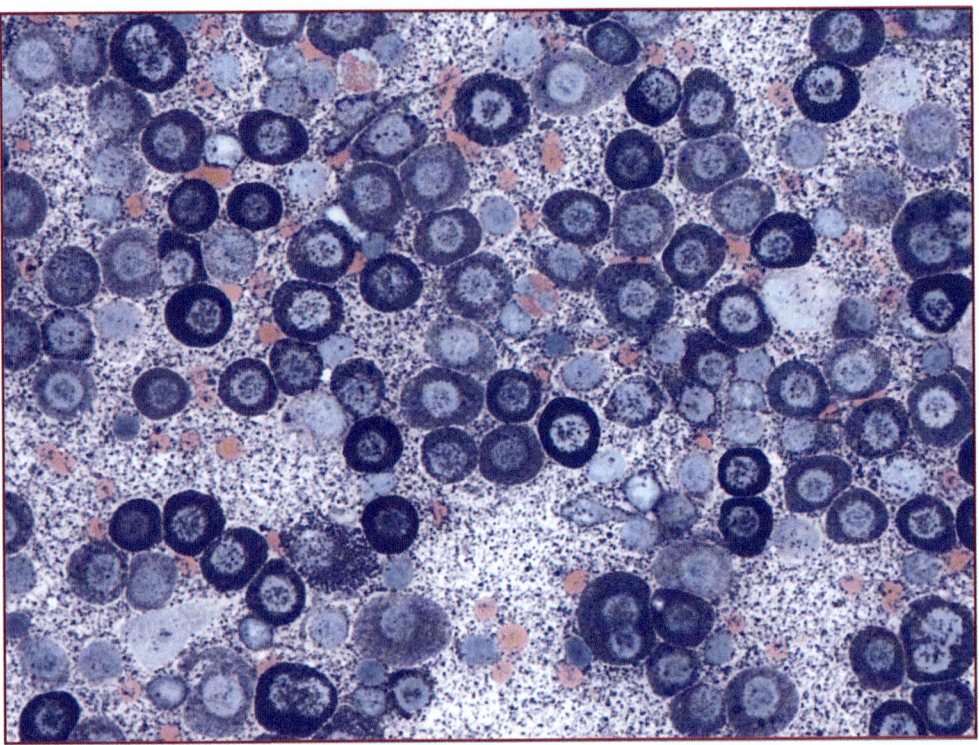

**Fig. 10.6.** Cat. Mast cell tumour. Wright-Giemsa.

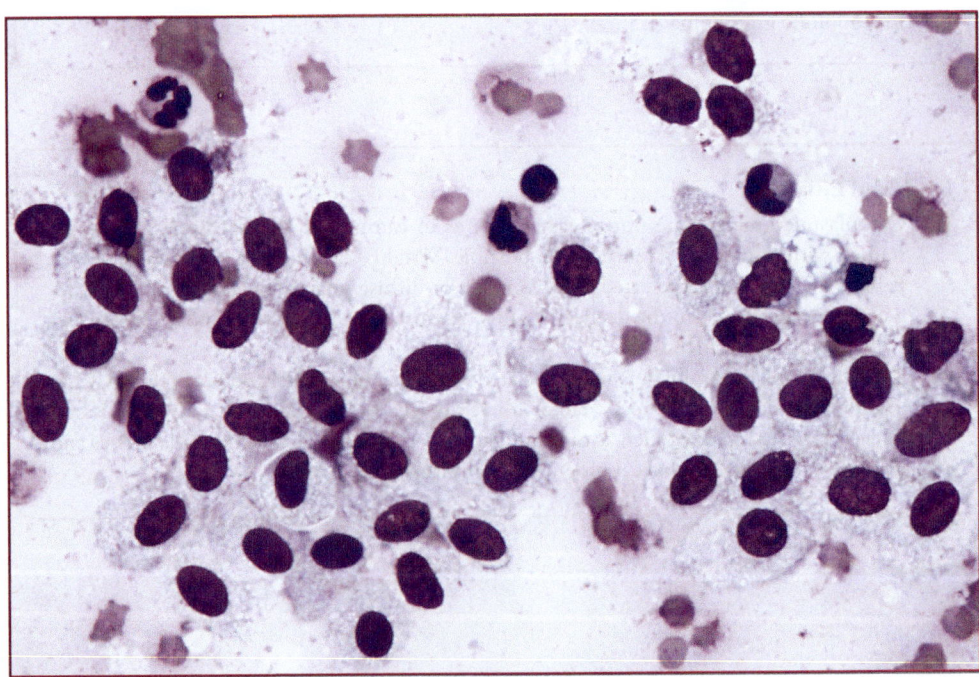

**Fig. 10.7.** Cat. Mast cell tumour, atypical histiocytic form. Wright-Giemsa. (*Courtesy of Robin Allison, Oklahoma State University.*)

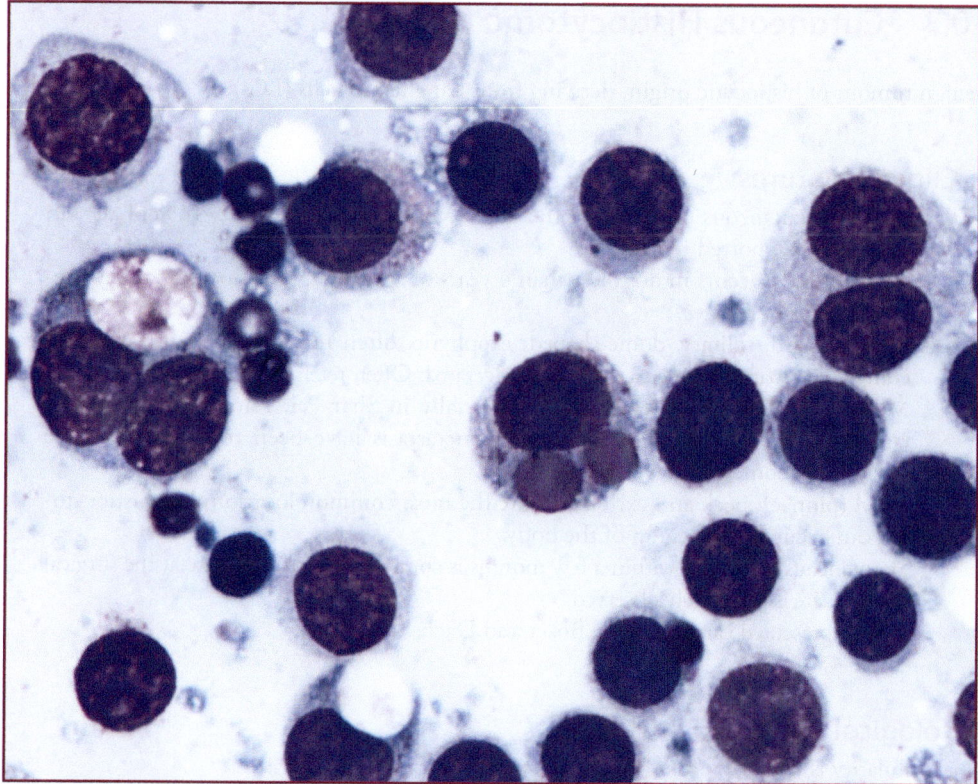

**Fig. 10.8.** Cat. Mast cell tumour. Mast cells are poorly granulated and often appear binucleated. Rarely they also show erythrophagocytosis. Wright-Giemsa. (*Courtesy of Erica Corda. Michigan State University, USA.*)

# Reference and further reading

Blackwood, L., Murphy, S., Buracco, P., De Vos, J.P., De Fornel-Thibaud, P., Hirschberger, J., Kessler, M., Pastor, J., Ponce, P., Savary-Bataille, K. *et al.* (2012) European consensus document on mast cell tumours in dogs and cats. *Veterinary Comparative Oncology* 10(3), 1–29.

Ho, N.T., Smith, K.C. and Dobromylskyj, M.J. (2018) Retrospective study of more than 9000 feline cutaneous tumours in the UK. *Journal of Feline Medicine and Surgery* 20(2), 128–134.

Kiupel, M. (2016) Mast cell tumours. In: Meuten, D.J. (ed.) *Tumors in Domestic Animals*, 5th edn. Wiley Blackwell, Ames, Iowa, pp. 176–202.

Melville, K., Smith, K.C. and Dobromylskyj, M.J. (2015) Feline cutaneous mast cell tumours: a UK-based study comparing signalment and histological features with long-term outcomes. *Journal of Feline Medicine and Surgery* 17(6), 486–493.

Piviani, M., Walton, R.M. and Patel, R.T. (2013) Significance of mastocytemia in cats. *Veterinary Clinical Pathology* 42(1), 4–10.

Sabattini, S. and Bettini, G. (2018) Grading cutaneous mast cell tumours in cats. *Veterinary Pathology*, early view (epub ahead of print).

## 10.3   Cutaneous Histiocytoma (Dog)

Benign tumour of histiocytic origin, deriving from Langherans cells (LCs).

### Clinical features
- Common cutaneous neoplasm of the dog, accounting for about 12–14% of all skin masses. Not reported in cats.
- Age: it mostly occurs in dogs less than 4 years of age, though histiocytoma may present in dogs of all ages.
- Variably sized, solitary, dome-shaped, exophytic, often red, cutaneous masses with complete or partial alopecia and often ulcerated. Often referred to as 'button' tumour. Multiple nodules have been reported, especially in Shar Pei. Rare cases of solitary cutaneous histiocytoma with lymph node metastasis have been reported and have variable outcomes.
- Head (pinnae), neck and extremities are the most common locations but histiocytoma can occur in any region of the body.
- Spontaneous regression within a few months is common. Recurrence rate at the surgical excision site is only rarely observed.
- Over-represented canine breeds: Boxer and Dachshund.

### Cytological features
- Cellularity is variable, often high.
- Background: often basophilic and variably haemodiluted.
- Neoplastic cells are round to oval, occasionally with small cytoplasmic projections and variably distinct cytoplasmic borders. They exfoliate individually.
- Nuclei are round, oval or reniform. They are often indented, paracentral to eccentric and have finely stippled chromatin. Single or multiple round nucleoli are frequently seen.
- The cytoplasm is moderate in amount, lightly basophilic, often lighter than the surrounding background. It may contain rare clear vacuoles and at times it may be wispy and paler at the outer edge of the cells.
- Cytological pleomorphism is variable to moderate. Anisocytosis and anisokaryosis are mild to moderate; binucleated cells and mitotic figures can be present.
- Small lymphocytes are often observed in the regressing phase of the tumour and may become the predominant cell type.

#### Differential diagnoses
- Large cell lymphoma
- Plasma cell tumour
- Small cell lymphoma (in regressing forms)

**Pearls and Pitfalls**

- Cytologically, cutaneous histiocytoma may sometimes resemble other round cell tumours, including large cell lymphoma and plasma cell tumour. Histopathology and immunohistochemical studies may help to provide a definitive diagnosis.
- Regressing cutaneous histiocytoma is accompanied by a progressive lymphocytic infiltrate (CD8+ T-cells). In the later stages, this may be difficult to differentiate from a cutaneous small cell lymphoma. In these cases, molecular clonality testing (PARR) might be considered to assist in the diagnosis. However, clonal T-cell expansions have been documented in association with the cytotoxic T-cell response to histiocytoma.

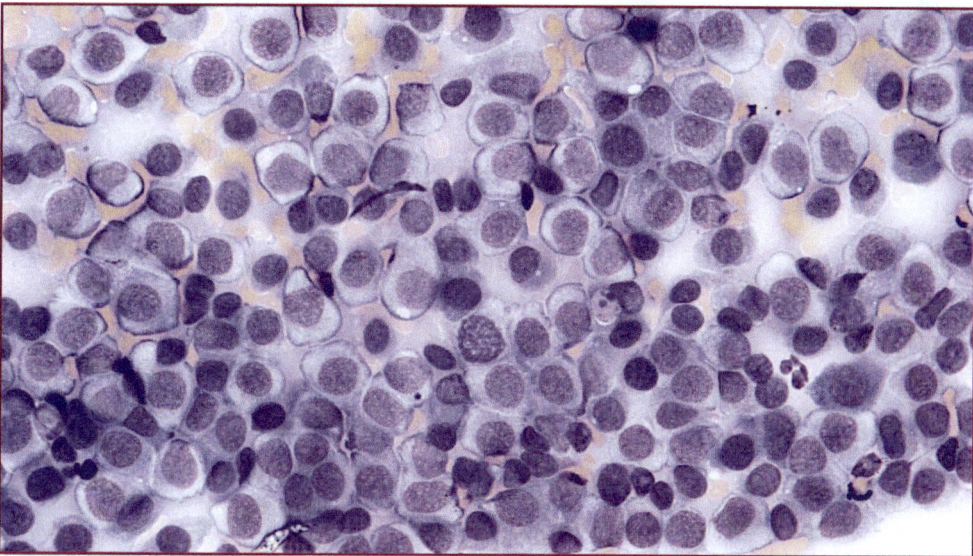

**Fig. 10.9.** Dog. Cutaneous histiocytoma. Wright-Giemsa.

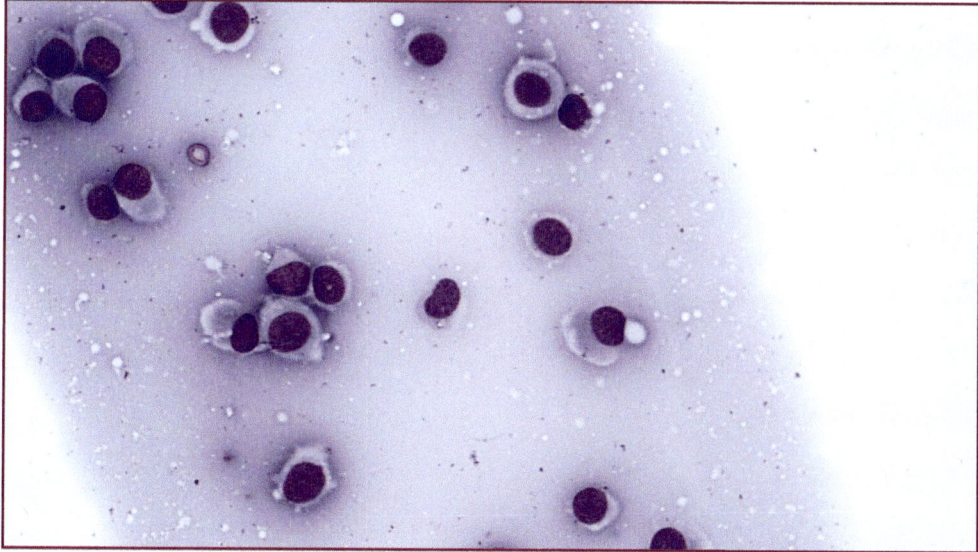

**Fig. 10.10.** Dog. Cutaneous histiocytoma. The cytoplasm of the histiocytes is lighter than the surrounding background. Wright-Giemsa.

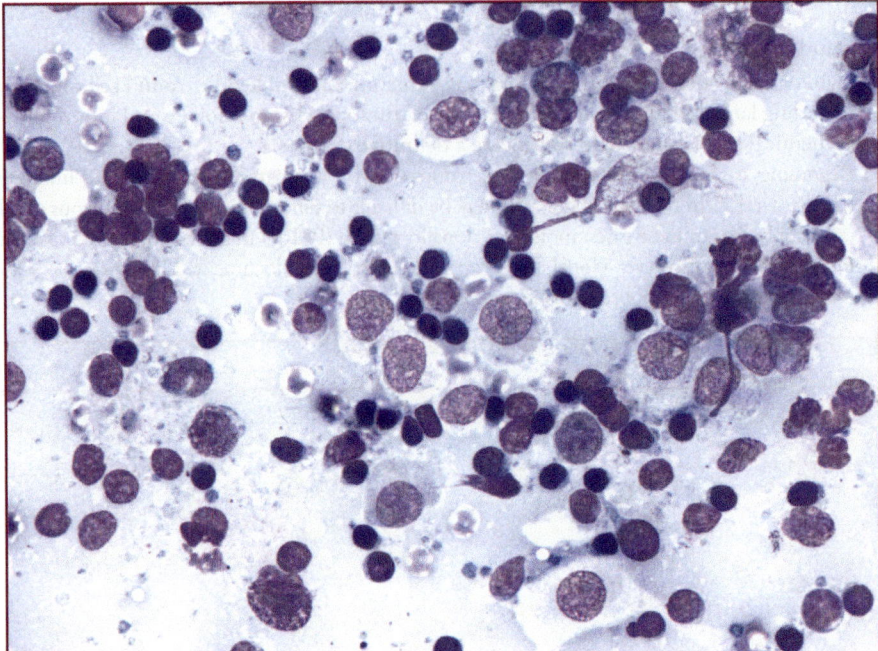

**Fig. 10.11.** Dog. Regressing cutaneous histiocytoma. Small lymphocytes admixed with histiocytes. Wright-Giemsa.

## Further reading

Faller, M., Lamm, C., Affolter, V.K., Valerius, K., Schwartz, S. and Moore, P.F. (2016) Retrospective characterisation of solitary cutaneous histiocytoma with lymph node metastasis in eight dogs. *Journal of Small Animal Practice* 57(10), 548–552.

Moore, P.F. (2014) A review of histiocytic diseases of dogs and cats. *Veterinary Pathology* 51(1), 167–184.

## 10.4   Plasma Cell Tumour

Benign tumour of plasma cells, also known as plasmacytoma.

### Clinical features

- Common cutaneous neoplasm of the dog, accounting for approximately 2% of all canine skin tumours. Only rarely reported in the cat.
- It mostly occurs in older dogs, with an average age of approximately 10 years old.
- Small, single, slightly raised dermal nodules, covered by alopecic and occasionally ulcerated skin. Multiple forms are rare but have also been reported in the absence of multiple myeloma. These are referred to as cutaneous plasmacytosis.
- Pinnae and digits are the common locations but oral cavity may also be affected in dogs. In cats, they have been documented on paws, thorax, face (lip, chin), neck, shoulder, tail, metatarsus and nose.
- The clinical behaviour is usually benign in dogs. Recurrence after complete surgical excision, metastases to distant skin sites and peripheral blood involvement have all been reported on rare occasions.
- In cats, less is known about the clinical behaviour of this tumour, due to the paucity of reported cases in the literature. For forms localized to the skin and/or regional lymph node, surgical excision usually guarantees long-term disease control. Early progression to systemic disease is reported in a few cases.
- Over-represented canine breeds: Yorkshire Terrier, Airedale Terrier, Kerry Blue Terrier, Scottish Terrier, Cocker Spaniel and Standard Poodle.

### Cytological features

- Cellularity is variable, often high.
- Background: clear or pale basophilic, variably haemodiluted.
- Plasma cells are round to oval with a moderate N:C ratio.
- Most of the time cells exfoliate individually, but occasionally they can form cluster-like arrangements.
- Nuclei are generally round, occasionally oval and eccentric. The chromatin is uniform to slightly clumped and nucleoli are indistinct.
- The cytoplasm is moderate to abundant and moderately to deeply basophilic. It may contain a perinuclear clearing in the area of the Golgi zone. Russel bodies (inclusions containing immunoglobulin) may be found in some of the cells.
- Rarely, very fine needle-like inclusions (Auer-like bodies) or blue–black fine granules of iron may be observed.
- Pleomorphism is variable and may be marked. Anisocytosis, anisokaryosis, bi- and/or multinucleation can be marked. In these cases, neoplastic cells often lose their distinctive features of typical plasma cells.
- Amyloid has been sporadically observed in a small percentage of well-differentiated plasma cell tumours. Cytologically, amyloid appears as extracellular pink amorphous material, which stains red–orange with Congo red. Amyloid can elicit a granulomatous inflammatory response with multinucleated giant cells.
- Erythrophagocytosis by neoplastic plasma cells has rarely been reported.

**Differential diagnoses**
- Lymphoma
- Cutaneous histiocytoma (in dogs)
- Peripheral nerve sheath tumour (in cats)
- Amelanotic melanoma (when poorly differentiated/granulated)
- Extraskeletal osteosarcoma

**Pearls and Pitfalls**
- Morphological features are not predictive of the biological behaviour and also markedly pleomorphic plasma cell tumours have a benign behaviour. However, the more atypia is present, the more difficult it is to differentiate this tumour from other neoplasms. In these cases, immunocyto/histochemical studies may help in reaching a definitive diagnosis. Plasma cells are often positive to MUM1 and, in a variable percentage of cases, to other B-cell markers (e.g. CD79a, CD20).
- When in doubt between plasma cell tumour and histiocytoma, the presence of prominent anisokaryosis and multinucleation is considered more supportive of plasma cell tumour.

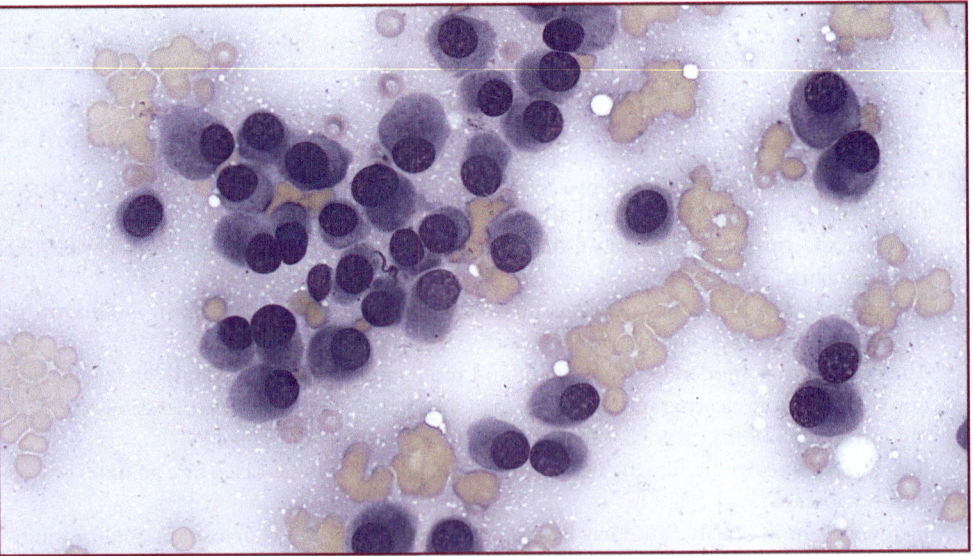

**Fig. 10.12.** Dog. Plasma cell tumour. Wright-Giemsa.

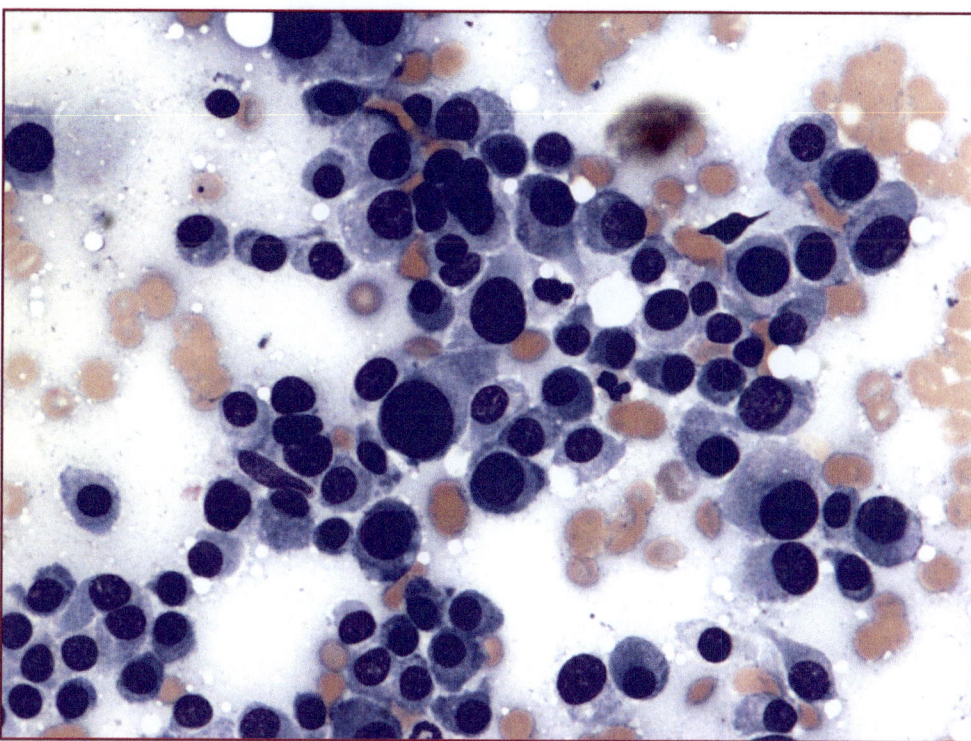

**Fig. 10.13.** Dog. Plasma cell tumour with prominent anisokaryosis. Wright-Giemsa.

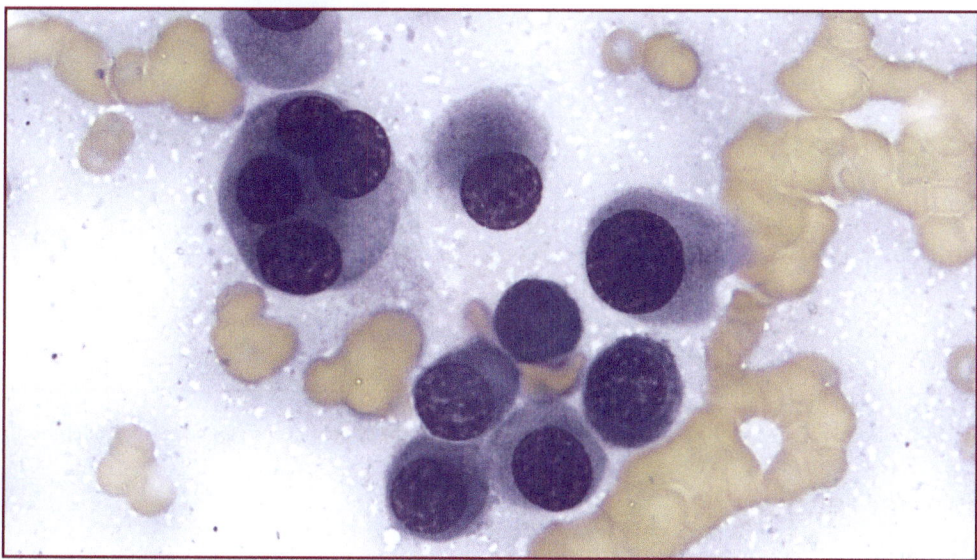

**Fig. 10.14.** Dog. Plasma cell tumour with multinucleated cells. Wright-Giemsa.

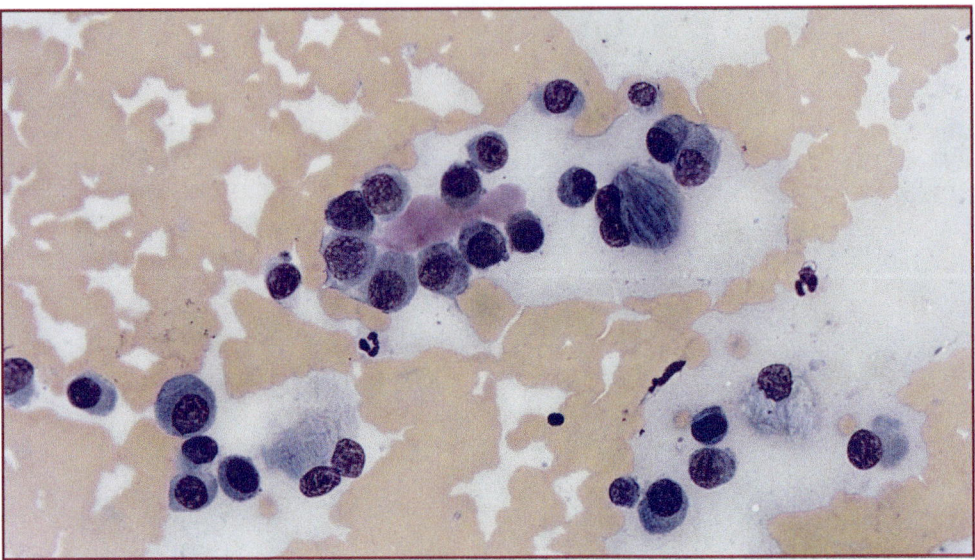

**Fig. 10.15.** Dog. Plasma cell tumour. Some of the cells surround a small amount of bright pink amorphous material (amyloid). Note that some of the neoplastic cells contain elongated Russel bodies (Mott cells). Wright-Giemsa.

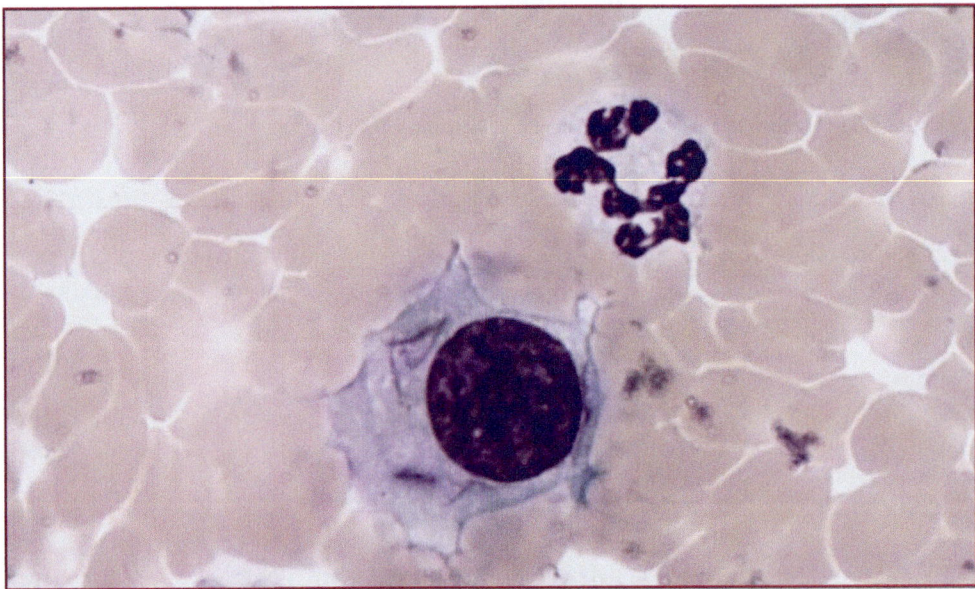

**Fig. 10.16.** Dog. Plasma cell tumour. Auer bodies can be seen within the cytoplasm of a plasma cell. Wright-Giemsa.

# Further reading

Boostrom, B.O., Moore, A.S., DeRegis, C.J., Robat, C., Freeman, K. and Thamm, D.H. (2017) Canine cutaneous plasmacytosis: 21 cases (2005–2015). *Journal of Veterinary Internal Medicine* 31(4), 1074–1080.

Quiroz-Rocha, G.F., Deravi, N. and Knight, B. (2017) What is your diagnosis? A pigmented round cell tumor. *Veterinary Clinical Pathology* 46(3), 538–539.

Tremblay, N., Lanevschi, A., Dore, M., Lanthier, I. and Desnovers, M. (2005) Of all the nerve! A subcutaneous forelimb mass on a cat. *Veterinary Clinical Pathology* 34(4), 417–420.

# 10.5   Transmissible Venereal Tumour (TVT)

Largely benign, contagious venereal neoplasm of probable histiocytic lineage. It is also known as Sticker's sarcoma.

## Clinical features

- Cutaneous neoplasm occurring in intact stray and wild dogs that exhibit unrestrained sexual activity. It is transmitted most commonly by coitus.
- It can develop at any age.
- Variably sized, cauliflower-like, pedunculated, nodular, papillary or multilobulated masses, firm but friable. The surface is often ulcerated and infected.
- Almost always located on the external genitalia; it may also occur in adjacent skin and oral, nasal and conjunctival mucosae.
- Spontaneous regression within a few months is common.
- Prognosis is generally good. Metastatic spread is occasionally described, in which case the prognosis is poorer. Metastasis is usually observed in dogs with compromised immunocompetency.

## Cytological features

- Cellularity is variable, often high.
- Background: often basophilic and variably haemodiluted.
- Neoplastic cells are round and discrete with distinct cytoplasmic borders.
- Nuclei are almost perfectly round, paracentral to eccentric, with coarse chromatin. Single or multiple round nucleoli may be seen.
- The cytoplasm is moderate to abundant and lightly basophilic. It often contains punctate clear vacuoles. These are often located along the cell borders.
- Cytological features of atypia are variable, up to moderate. They include anisocytosis, anisokaryosis and presence of mitotic figures.
- Small lymphocytes are often observed in the regressing phase. Reactive fibroblasts associated with collagen bundles may also be found.
- Neutrophils may be present in ulcerated lesions.

### Differential diagnoses
- Other round cell tumours
- Amelanotic melanoma

### Pearls and Pitfalls

If the tumour arises deep in the prepuce or vagina, it may be difficult to find without careful physical examination; this may lead to misdiagnosis if bleeding is confounded with oestrus, urethritis, cystitis or prostatitis.

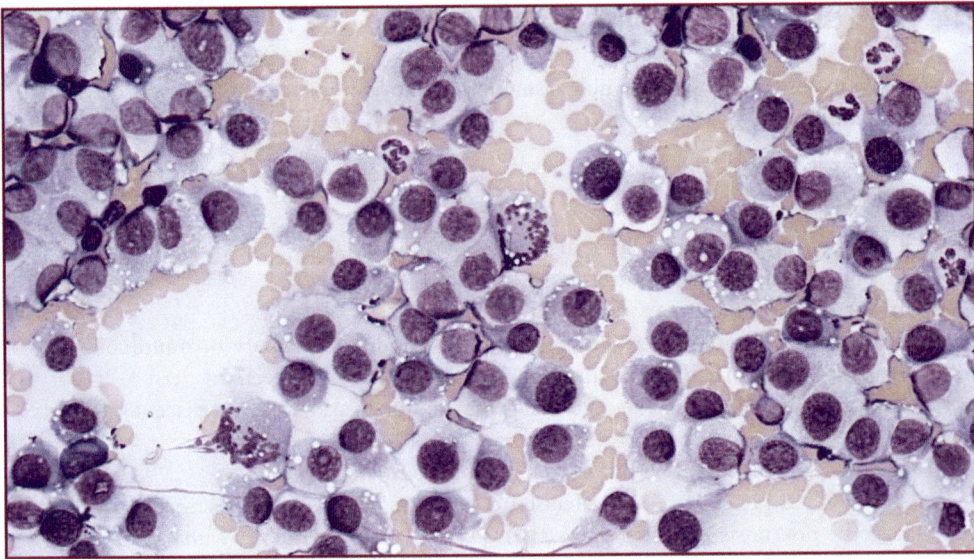

**Fig. 10.17.** Dog. TVT. Wright-Giemsa.

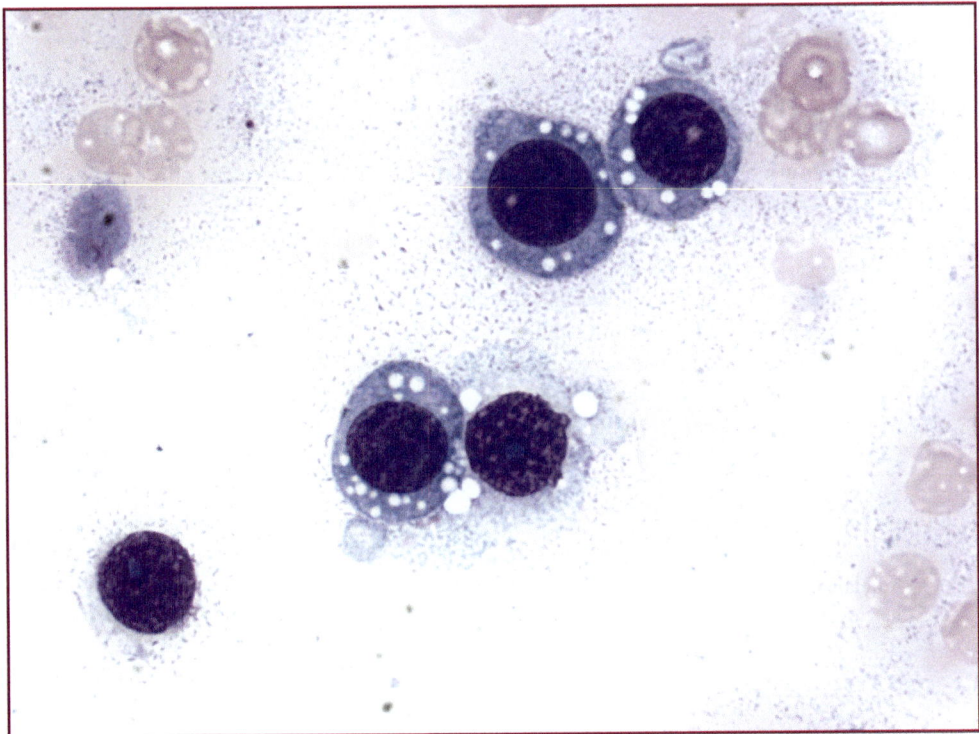

**Fig. 10.18.** Dog. TVT. Note the clear punctate vacuoles arranged in an orderly manner around the cytoplasm borders. Wright-Giemsa.

## Further reading

Ganguly, B., Das, U. and Das, A.K. (2013) Canine transmissible venereal tumour; a review. *Veterinary Comparative Oncology* 14(1), 1–12.

# 10.6   Cutaneous Lymphoma

Primary lymphoproliferative disease infiltrating the epidermis and/or cutaneous adnexa (epithe-liotropic lymphoma) or the dermis (cutaneous non-epitheliotropic lymphoma).

## Clinical features

- Uncommon cutaneous neoplasm of the dog and the cat, accounting for about 1% and up to 2.8% of all skin tumours in dogs and cats, respectively.
- Age: it mostly occurs in older animals, with an average age of approximately 10 years old in both species.
- The clinical presentation is variable and non-specific and could mimic other dermatopa-thies. It may occur in the form of single or multiple nodules, plaques, ulcers, erythaemic or exfoliative dermatitis, often covered by scaly plaques with focal hypopigmentation and alopecia. In dogs, lesions are often pruritic. Mucocutaneous forms may involve the gums, lips and anal mucosa. These often appear thick, ulcerated and inflamed.
- In advanced stages, peripheral lymph nodes, internal organs, peripheral blood and/or bone marrow may be involved. When neoplastic lymphoid cells appear in the blood, the condition is called *Sezary syndrome*.
- Over-represented canine breeds: Cocker Spaniel, Bulldog, Boxer, Scottish Terrier and Golden Retriever.
- Cutaneous epitheliotropic lymphoma (CETL):
  - T-cell (CD8+) immunophenotype.
  - It is the most common form of cutaneous lymphoma in dogs. It is extremely rare in cats.
  - Neoplastic cells show affinity for the epithelial cells of the epidermis and adnexal structures. If they are confined above the basement membrane of the epidermis or the epithelium of adnexa, the disease is referred to as *pagetoid reticulosis*. This form is not very common in the dog and cat. When the neoplastic cells involve both the epithelium of the skin and the dermis, the form is known as *mycosis fungoides* (from the mushroom-like appearance of the lesions).
- Cutaneous non-epitheliotropic lymphoma (NEL):
  - T- or B-cell immunophenotype.
  - Non-epitheliotropic lymphoma is the most common form of cutaneous lymph-oma in cats; it is uncommon in dogs.
  - Neoplastic cells are localized in the dermis with no involvement of the epidermis and/or adnexa.
- Cutaneous lymphoma at injection sites (CLIS) is an uncommon form of non-epitheliotropic lymphoma that has been reported in cats in the setting of sub-acute to chronic inflammation induced by injections. Due to this, it is more common in the lateral thorax and interscapular regions. Reported cases mostly have a B-cell immunopheno-type and show marked angiotropism.
- A subcutaneous panniculitis-like T-cell lymphoma (SPTCL) has also been described in dogs. In this type of lymphoma, the neoplastic cells selectively involve the subcutis.
- Little is known about the clinical behaviour of cutaneous lymphoma. However, the non-epitheliotropic lymphoma seems to be more aggressive and more rapidly pro-gressive than the epitheliotropic form.

## Cytological features

- Cellularity is variable, often high.
- Background: often clear and variably haemodiluted. It may contain small cytoplasmic fragments (lymphoglandular bodies).
- Epitheliotropic lymphoma: most frequently composed of small- to medium-sized lymphoid cells. Mitoses are rare or absent. Less commonly, neoplastic cells are medium-large, with high mitotic activity.
- Non-epitheliotropic lymphoma: neoplastic cells are often large with high numbers of mitoses. NEL composed by a predominance of small lymphocytes has also been observed. Small cell forms have also been observed.
- Small cell forms:
  - Nuclei are small to intermediate (< 1.5 rbc), round, often indented, irregular and cerebriform. They have a finely clumped chromatin and small nucleoli can be seen.
  - The cytoplasm is scant to moderate and pale basophilic.
  - Mitoses are usually absent, or present in very low numbers.
- Large cell forms:
  - Nuclei are large (> 2.5 rbc), round, often convoluted and indented, with coarse granular chromatin and prominent nucleoli.
  - The cytoplasm is moderate in amount and variably basophilic.
  - Marked nuclear pleomorphism and binucleation have been reported. Mitoses can be numerous and atypical.
- Inflammatory cells are frequently present. A neutrophilic and macrophagic inflammation is often observed secondary to ulceration of the lesions. Secondary opportunistic bacterial infection can develop. In the non-epitheliotropic lymphoma, an infiltrate of histiocytes, neutrophils and mixed lymphocytes can accompany the neoplastic component (inflammatory NEL), making the diagnosis of a lymphoma more difficult.

---

**Differential diagnoses**
- Small cell lymphoma:
  - Lymphocytic (chronic) inflammation
  - Regressing cutaneous histiocytoma
- Large cell lymphoma:
  - Histiocytic neoplasm (e.g. cutaneous histiocytoma, histiocytic sarcoma and reactive histiocytosis)
  - Mixed inflammatory dermatitis
- Subcutaneous panniculitis-like T-cell lymphoma:
  - Panniculitis

**Pearls and Pitfalls**

- Definitive diagnosis of cutaneous lymphoma may require additional testing, including histopathology ideally accompanied by immunophenotypical techniques (immunohistochemistry, flow cytometry) and/or clonality assay (PARR – PCR for antigen receptor rearrangement). This is particularly useful in the small cell forms, which may appear undistinguishable from lymphocytic inflammation.
- Cutaneous lymphoma can also be the manifestation of a generalized form of lymphoma.

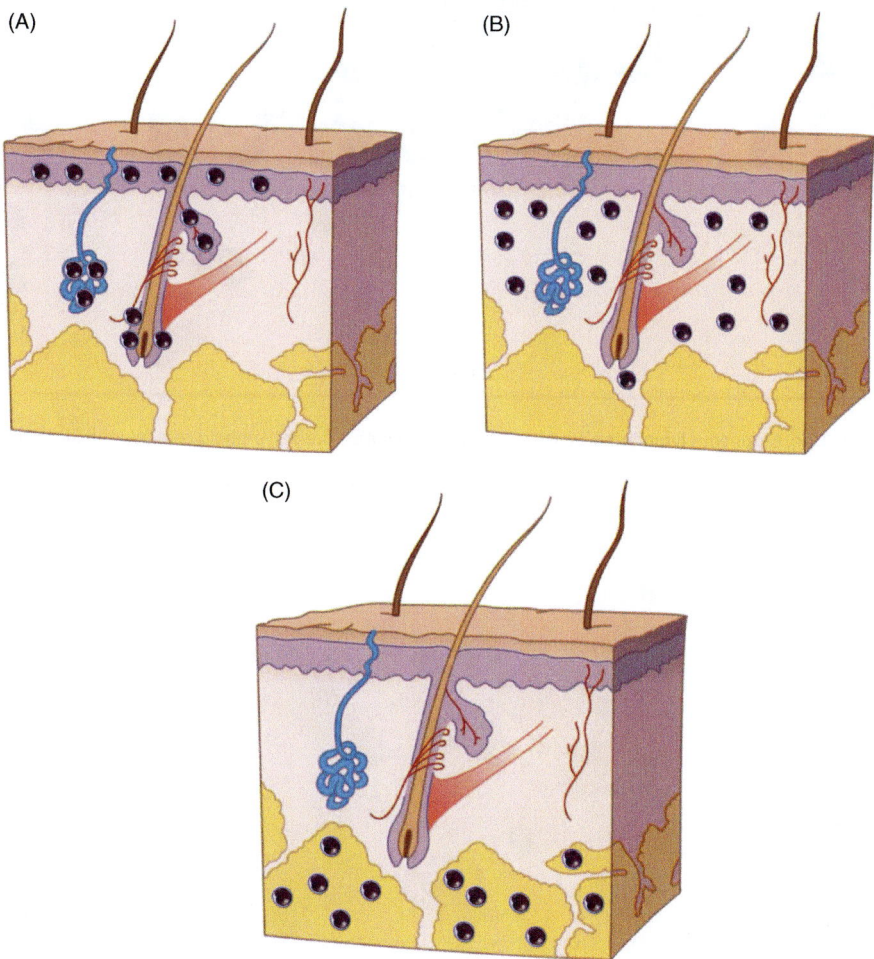

**Fig. 10.19.** Schematic representation of the distribution of neoplastic lymphoid cells in (A) cutaneous epitheliotropic lymphoma, (B) cutaneous non-epitheliotropic lymphoma and (C) subcutaneous lymphoma.

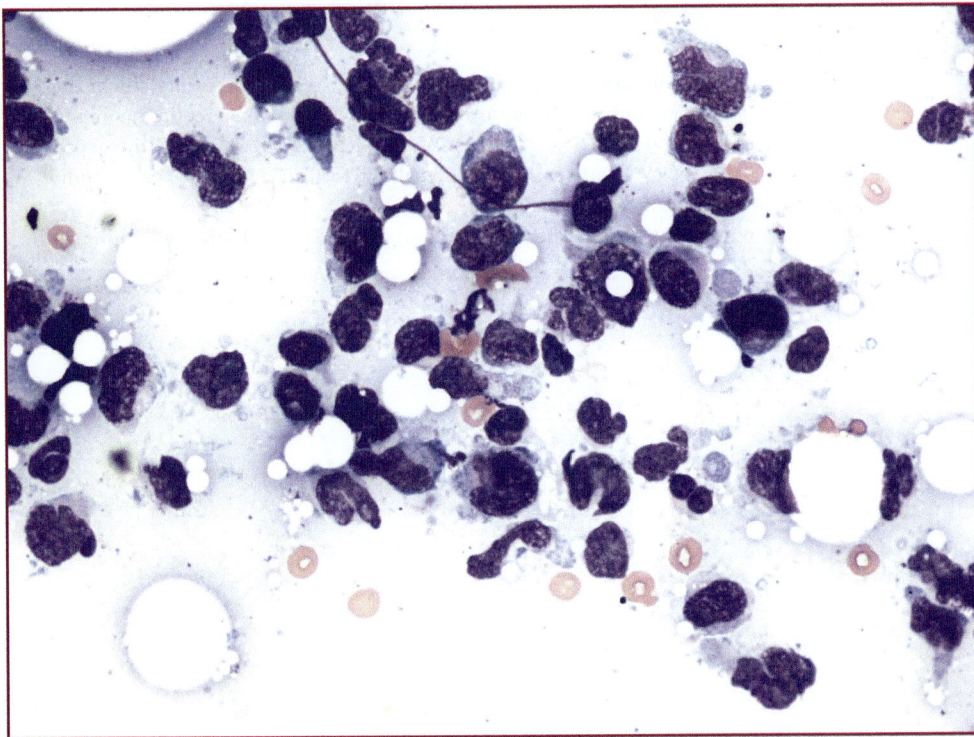

**Fig. 10.20.** Dog. Cutaneous lymphoma. Pleomorphic, intermediate to large lymphoid cells. Wright-Giemsa.

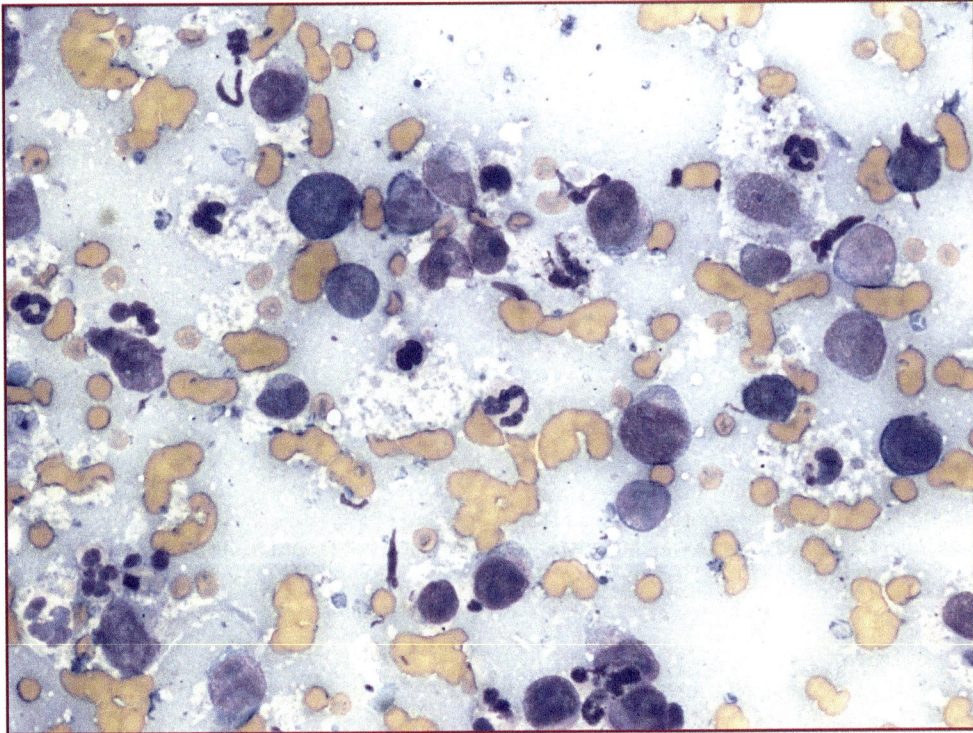

**Fig. 10.21.** Cat. Cutaneous lymphoma. Large lymphoid cells admixed with a few blood-derived leucocytes. Wright-Giemsa.

# Further reading

Fontaine, J., Bovens, C., Bettenay, S. and Mueller, R.S. (2009) Canine cutaneous epitheliotropic T-cell lymphoma: a review. *Veterinary Comparative Oncology* 7(1), 1–14.

Fontaine, J., Heimann, M. and Day, M.J. (2011) Canine cutaneous epitheliotropic T-cell lymphoma: a review of 30 cases. *Veterinary Dermatology* 21(3), 267–275.

Fontaine, J., Heimann, M. and Day, M.J. (2011) Cutaneous epitheliotropic T-cell lymphoma in the cat: a review of the literature and five new cases. *Veterinary Dermatology* 22(5), 454–461.

Noland, E.L., Keller, S.M. and Kiupel, M. (2018) Subcutaneous panniculitis-like T-cell lymphoma in dogs: Morphologic and immunohistochemical classification. *Veterinary Pathology* 55(6), 802–808.

Roccabianca, P., Avallone, G., Rodriguez, A., Crippa, L., Lepri, E., Giudice, C., Caniatti, M., Moore, P.F. and Affolter, V.K. (2016) Cutaneous lymphoma at injection sites: pathological, immunophenotypical, and molecular characterization in 17 cats. *Veterinary Pathology* 53(4), 823–832.

Rook, K.A. (2019) Canine and feline cutaneous epitheliotropic lymphoma and cutaneous lymphocytosis. *Veterinary Clinics of North America Small Animal Practice* 49(1), 67–81.

# 11 Metastatic Lesions

## General information

Skin metastases of non-primary skin tumours are extremely rare in dogs and cats and only sporadic cases have been reported in the literature. In certain cases, cutaneous metastases may be the first sign of an undiagnosed non-cutaneous malignancy. An accurate search for a primary disease, knowledge of any previous history of neoplasia and the awareness of certain established tumour patterns of metastases (e.g. metastatic bronchial carcinoma to the digits in cats) are crucial to help in establishing the nature of the metastatic process, as cytology alone may not be sufficient. Cutaneous metastases have been reported for the following neoplasms:

- Epithelial tumours:
  - Gastrointestinal carcinoma (dogs, cats).
  - Renal carcinoma (dogs).
  - Transitional cell carcinoma (dogs).
  - Pulmonary carcinoma (including the lung–digit syndrome of cats).
  - Mammary carcinoma (including inflammatory mammary carcinoma in dogs).
  - Neuroendocrine carcinoma of nasal origin (dogs).
- Mesenchymal tumours:
  - Haemangiosarcoma (dogs).
  - Rhabdomyosarcoma (dogs).
  - Osteosarcoma (dogs).
- Round cell tumours:
  - Visceral mast cell tumour (dogs and cats).
  - Multiple myeloma (dogs).
  - Transmissible venereal tumour (dogs).
- Sex cord stromal tumours:
  - Seminoma (dogs).
  - Leydig cell tumour (dogs).

Lymphoma and histiocytic neoplasms arising from other organs may also secondarily involve the skin, as progression of a generalized disease.

## Cytological features

- The cytological features of the tumours listed above are typical of the primary neoplasm. The reader should refer to specific cytology textbooks for detailed morphological descriptions.

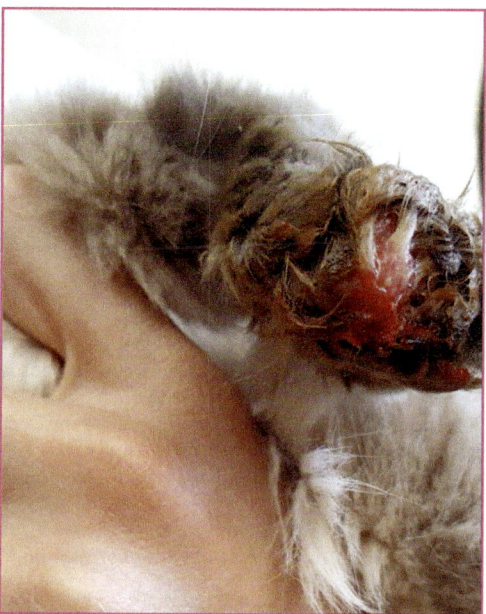

**Fig. 11.1.** Cat. Ulceration and onychomadesis of a digit with metastatic bronchogenic carcinoma to the digit. (*Courtesy of Raqueli Teresinha Franca.*)

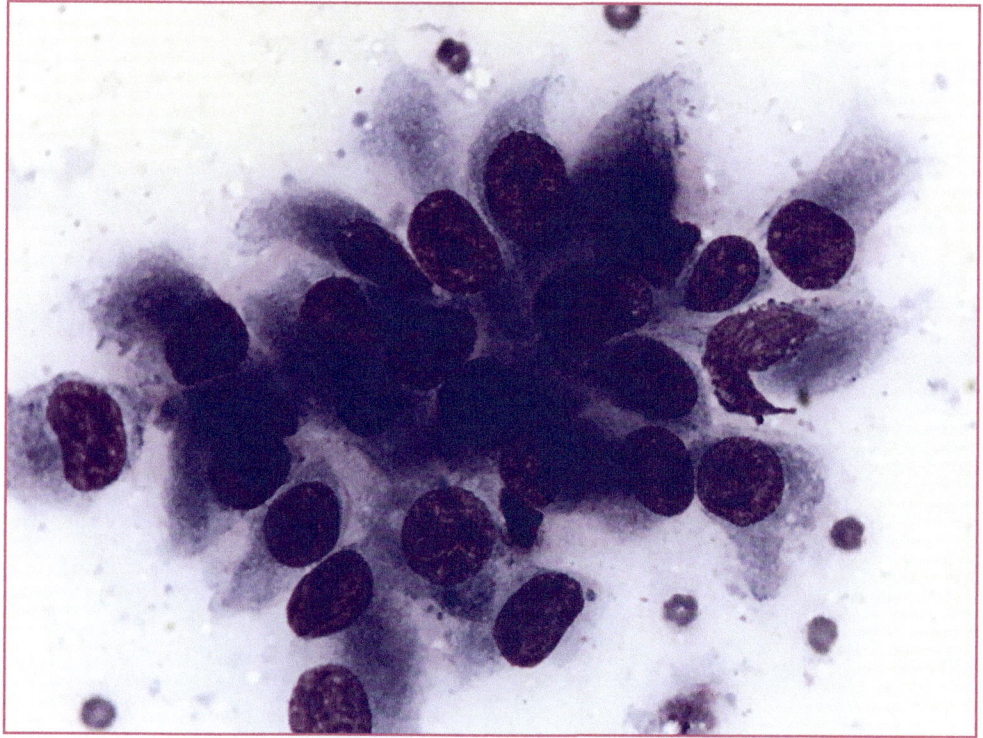

**Fig. 11.2.** Cat. Metastatic bronchial carcinoma (lung–digit syndrome). Cluster of columnar bronchial cells with moderate anisokaryosis and prominent nucleoli. Wright-Giemsa. (*Courtesy of Raqueli Teresinha Franca.*)

# 12 Suggested Further Reading and References

Goldschmidt, M.H., Munday, J.S., Scruggs, J.L., Klopfleisch, R. and Kiupel, M. (2018) *Surgical Pathology of Tumors of Domestic Animals, Volume 1: Epithelial Tumors of the Skin*. Davis-Thompson DVM Foundation, Gurnee, Illinois.

Gross, T.L., Ihrke, P.J., Walder, E.J. and Affolter, V.K. (2005) *Skin Diseases of the Dog and Cat: Clinical and Histo-pathologic Diagnosis*, 2nd edn. Blackwell Science, Ames, Iowa.

Maxie, M.G. (2016) *Jubb, Kennedy and Palmer's Pathlogy of Domestic Animals*, 6th edn. Saunders, St Louis, Missouri.

Meuten, D.J. (ed.) (2017) *Tumors in Domestic Animals*, 5th edn. Wiley Blackwell, Ames, Iowa.

Valenciano, A.C. and Cowell, R.L. (2014) *Cowell and Tyler's Diagnostic Cytology and Hematology of the Dog and Cat*, 4th edn. Elsevier, St Louis, Missouri.

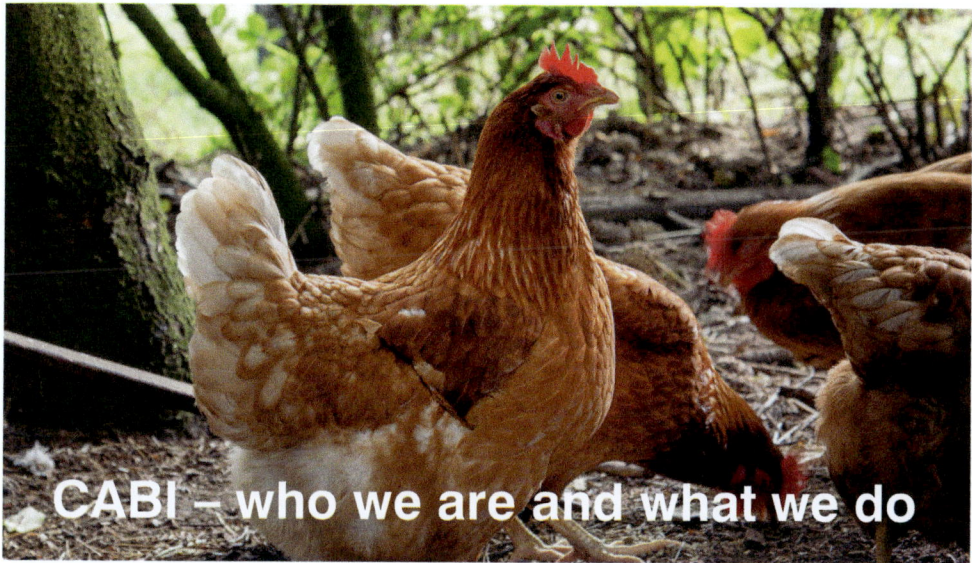

CABI – who we are and what we do

This book is published by **CABI**, an international not-for-profit organisation that improves people's lives worldwide by providing information and applying scientific expertise to solve problems in agriculture and the environment.

CABI is also a global publisher producing key scientific publications, including world renowned databases, as well as compendia, books, ebooks and full text electronic resources. We publish content in a wide range of subject areas including: agriculture and crop science / animal and veterinary sciences / ecology and conservation / environmental science / horticulture and plant sciences / human health, food science and nutrition / international development / leisure and tourism.

The profits from CABI's publishing activities enable us to work with farming communities around the world, supporting them as they battle with poor soil, invasive species and pests and diseases, to improve their livelihoods and help provide food for an ever growing population.

CABI is an international intergovernmental organisation, and we gratefully acknowledge the core financial support from our member countries (and lead agencies) including:

   Ministry of Agriculture People's Republic of China   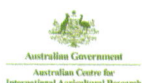 Australian Government Australian Centre for International Agricultural Research    Agriculture and Agri-Food Canada   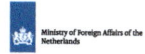 Ministry of Foreign Affairs of the Netherlands   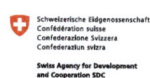 Schweizerische Eidgenossenschaft Confédération suisse Confederazione Svizzera Confederaziun svizra Swiss Agency for Development and Cooperation SDC

## Discover more

To read more about CABI's work, please visit: **www.cabi.org**

Browse our books at: **www.cabi.org/bookshop**,
or explore our online products at: **www.cabi.org/publishing-products**

Interested in writing for CABI? Find our author guidelines here:
**www.cabi.org/publishing-products/information-for-authors/**

Printed and bound by CPI Group (UK) Ltd, Croydon, CR0 4YY

23/04/2025

14661118-0005